THE ART
OF ZEN-TOUCH™

Seymour Koblin

FOREWORD

This book is written in two parts. The first section discusses the origins and fundamentals of Eastern healing concepts and Shiatsu. It offers a brief and simple explanation of both principle and practice. When readers feel comfortable with their understanding of Section I, it is my hope that the deeper experiential perspectives presented in Section II will be more easily assimilated.

After completing the book, I questioned some of the repetition existing within the two sections. I decided to leave it as is because I have consistently witnessed the value of repetition in my own learning. My greatest choice is that the *Art of Zen Touch*™ will enhance your path to health awareness and the communication of that experience with many others.

Many people have helped me in the writing of this book. I would like to extend special thanks to my teachers: Master CK Chu, Wataru Ohashi, Esther Turnbull, Michio Kushi, Shizuko Yamamoto, and my family and friends who motivated me to develop the *Art of Zen-Touch*™.

I am also most grateful to the following people and companies for their help in the production of this book:

Illustrations: Sharon Cadenhead Gould, Toni Meads, Kristi
                  Clark, Kavi Cornell, Greg and
                  Dan at Artifax, Joyce Beall and Nikki Badua.

Manuscript Typing
and Editing: Carol Dysart & Associates
                          Marcelle Evenska, Catherine Kineavy, Carla Boone,
                          Pam Greer, Shelby Simmers and Wendy Ruiz

Desktop Publishing: Joyce Beall, Sunwater Graphics

Photography: Suzette Lee/Positive Effects, Leslee Anglim,
                          Richard Spasoff and Carlos Richardson

Grounding Support: All Colleagues, Staff, Instructors and Friends, at the
                          School of Healing Arts, with special mention to Debbie
                          O'Connor, Gary de Rodriguez, Marilyn King, Kathy
                          Sheehy, Annie McGlone, Fafi Yousry, Pam Greer, Sheila
                          Steelman, and Shannon Thompson, who have supported
                          me with rooting, practicality, vision, patience and most
                          of all great love.

Zen Touch™
Interns and Instructors: Jeff St. Onge, Brett Brindley, Denise Nease, Erica
                          Tibbetts, Patti Pace, Melantha Tatum, Dave Garza, Hugo
                          Anguino, Leanne Tibiatowski, Rebecca Montoya,
                          Richard Ciaverelli, Tara Boyce, Thomas Curry, Delfina
                          Franco, Richard Goff, Benjamin Grunde, Beverly Kobie,
                          Erin McGibbon, Renate Nishio, K.R. Ridge, Chris Rizzi,
                          Carol Edwards, Stephanie Clark, Ross Landon, Kris
                          Trulock, and Fafi Yousry, whose trust in Zen-Touch™
                          makes me feel so humbly grateful.

                          In Gratitude
                          Infinitely ... Definitely

                          Seymour Koblin

TABLE OF CONTENTS

Continued...

Continued...

Part 1 - ASIAN BODY HEALING

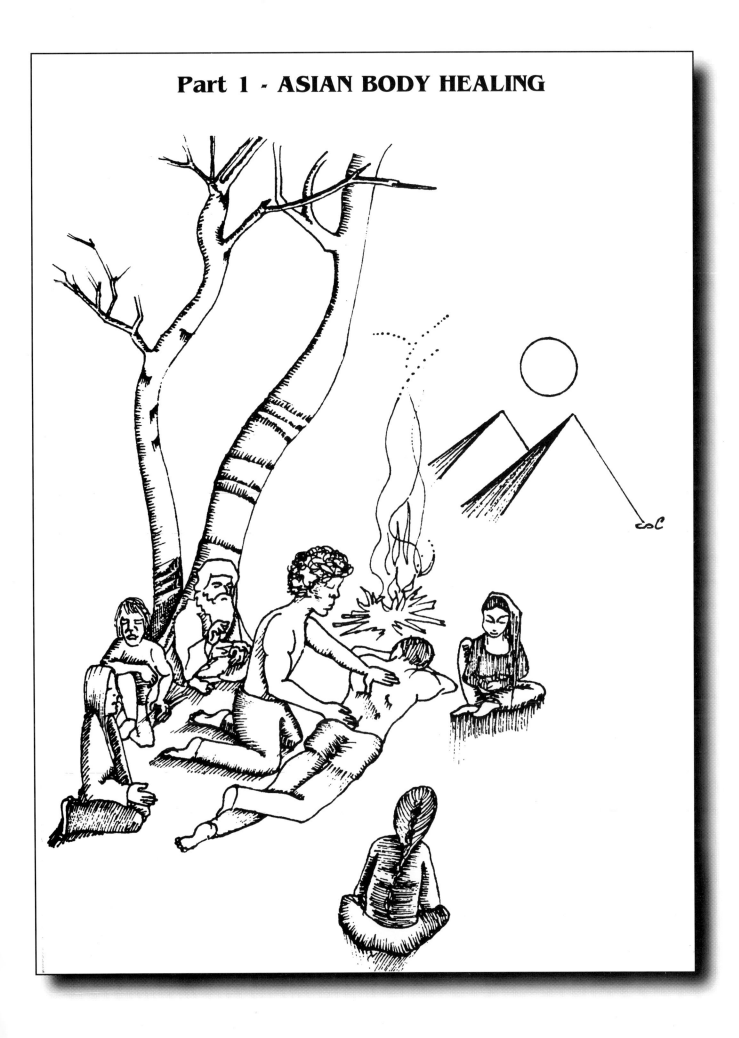

Part 1 - ASIAN BODY HEALING

Asian body healing originated thousands of years ago in the villages and small communities in and around the countries of India, China, Japan and Korea. The actual techniques used began as instinctive responses to manifestations of imbalance in the body. People frequently experienced comfort and relief from extreme sensations of tension, pain, heat and cold by touching body areas in different ways. Some people - *Healers* and *Shamans* - had an innate aptitude for initiating healing with others.

These founders of Asian massage and Meridian point therapy developed many styles that are practiced today. *Anma, Do-In, Reiki, Lomi Lomi, Marma Point Therapy, Tui Na, Jin Shin Jitsu, Acupressure and Shiatsu* are some of the better known styles. Human compassion was the motivating force behind traditional body healing, as practiced in the close-knit surroundings of the ancient villages. The welfare of family and friends was held with great reverence. Although the techniques have evolved a great deal since that time, it is important to emphasize that this attitude of love, respect and compassion for one's fellow beings provides the basis upon which the success of Asian body healing is dependent.

The people who dedicated themselves to healing knew very little about body mechanics. Their approach to illness lacked any knowledge of cells, muscles, nerves, physics, chemistry or biology. The only tools they utilized were their senses. They observed how the body reacted by means of sight, smell, sound, taste and intuition. Their **experience** became the foundation for assessment and therapy. Each person they worked with represented a microcosmic manifestation of the macrocosmic world, and everyone was treated individually, even if they displayed the same outward indications. Many aspects of a person's life-style including diet, climate, exercise, type of work, family relations and ancestral influences were considered relevant in order to ensure successful therapy. For example, if two people suffered from fatigue and one lived in a cold, mountainous region while the other came from a warmer island home, the methods utilized would have to be different for each of them. With respect to massage, the mountain dweller *might* have required a slower, more nurturing and tonifying style of work, while the island dweller *may* have benefited from a quick, invigorating of massage.

After working with many people over thousands of years, certain observations were collected on how all the elements of the environment harmoniously interweaved and coexisted with each other. Eventually, a system was devised to describe how the ever-changing forces of nature influenced the human body. This system was based on heaven's force originating from the constellations, interacting with the forces emanating from the earth. The former was called *yang* and the latter, *yin*. Heaven's yang force brought the rain, while earth's yin force responded with the growth of plants. The two were attracted to each other, creating a unity between complementary opposites: dark/light, hot/cold, expansion/contraction, moon/sun, woman/man. The relationship between these two natural forces was also applied to describe how energy flows through the body.

Understanding life through this system proved to be very effective, and the Yin/Yang theory, which originated in China, became the basis for most of the Asian healing arts. Simply stated, any imbalance or symptom ranging from a muscle pain to degenerative dis-ease can be identified as a distortion in the quantity and quality of the *yin* and *yang* forces.

Yang energy (heaven's force) enters the body through the crown of the head while *Yin* energy (earth's force) enters through the feet and lower torso. Because the two forces are attracted to each other, they collide, unite and complement each other along the body's central median plane. This energetic flow has been referred to as the *central, primary,* or *spiritual channel.* Many hours of intense internal exercise and meditation led to the formulation of theories that were based on experiencing this electric-like energy move through the body.

Through these experiences, it was also concluded that there were seven sources of energy vortexes along the central channel which were called the seven *Chakras.* (Figure 1, pg. 3). As earth's force and heaven's force converged at these locations, a series of secondary channels called *meridians* were generated that circulated away from the central channel (Figure 1, pg. 3). These meridians extended throughout the body nourishing the internal organs as well as providing the energy to activate all metabolic processes. The Chinese called this life-force energy *"chi."* Any disturbance in the flow of *chi* created imbalance in the body. The laws of physics and chemistry maintain that all phenomena exist in a balanced relationship between positively charged protons and their magnetic attraction to negatively charged electrons (Yang with Yin).

Also, movement of charged ions generates a flow of electromagnetic energy (called *chi*). Modern Quantum Physics states that the fundamental structure at the core of all life are forces of energy that are devoid of mass/weight. These forces are referred to as 1) gravity, 2) electromagnetic force, 3) the strong force which holds mass together, and 4) the weak force which disperses particles of mass. Alas, ancient eastern and modern western wisdom converge.

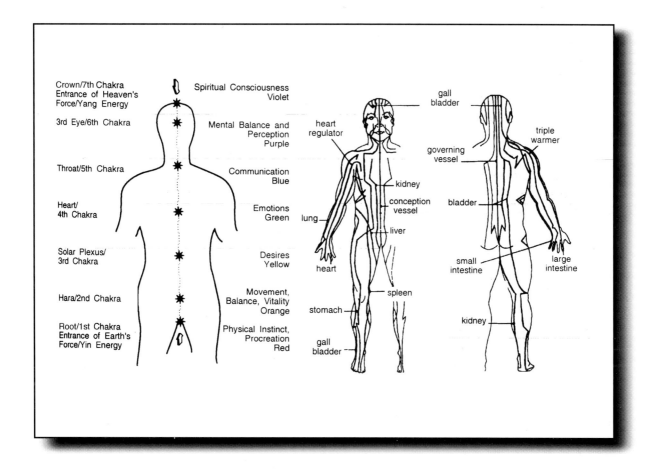

Figure 1

THE FIVE TRANSFORMATIONS

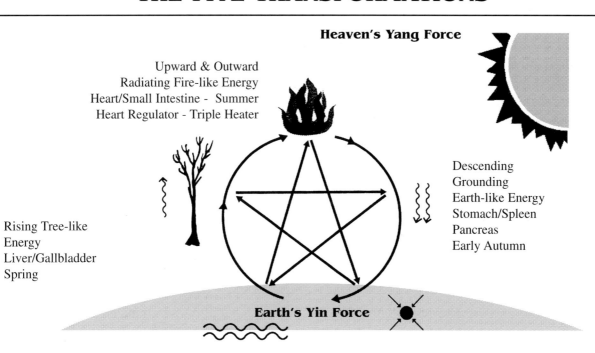

Heaven's Yang Force

Upward & Outward
Radiating Fire-like Energy
Heart/Small Intestine - Summer
Heart Regulator - Triple Heater

Descending
Grounding
Earth-like Energy
Stomach/Spleen
Pancreas
Early Autumn

Rising Tree-like
Energy
Liver/Gallbladder
Spring

Earth's Yin Force

	Flowing Cultivating Potential	Rising Sprouting Birth	Upward/outward Radiating Inspiration	Descending Grounding Nourishing	Gathering to Materialized Completion
Energy Movement:					
Elemental Example:	Water-like	Tree-like	Fire-like	Earth-like	Metal-like
Time:	Winter Night	Spring Morning	Summer Noon	Early Autumn Mid-afternoon	Fall Evening
Climatic Influence:	Cold	Windy	Hot	Humid	Dry
Body Organs & Meridians:	Kidneys, Bladder	Liver, Gallbladder	Heart Small Intestine Heart Regulator Triple Heater	Stomach, Spleen, Pancreas	Lungs, Large Intestine
Balanced Expression:	Courageous Flexible Positive	Patience Spontaneity	A Peaceful Charisma Sociable	Compassion Resourceful	Determination Dependable
Imbalanced Expression:	Fear Cautious	Frustration Anger	Mood Swings e.g., Hyper/depressed	Complainer	Stuck Stagnant

Figure 2

The meridians move through the body interweaving with each other, creating a web that assists and coordinates all body functions. Our physical, mental, emotional and spiritual condition are all influenced by the energy flowing through the meridians. For example, Asian healing professionals believe that the Kidney Meridian activates the kidneys to filter blood, and also plays an important role in assisting the body to adapt and flow through potentially stressful daily changes. Emotions like fear and the attitude of courage are associated with the   functions of the Kidney Meridian. All the meridian associations will be discussed later in this book.

When the totality of all life influences flowing through the meridians are balanced we experience vital health. Also, because the meridians move throughout the entire body, it is possible to correlate various body signals that lie on a meridian line (discoloration, pain, skin markings) with the physical and psychological attributes of that particular meridian. For example, if someone feels muscle tightness/pain in a certain area that corresponds with the Kidney Meridian line, a correlation may be discovered that links this physical symptom to an imbalance in the kidneys job of filtering blood as well as an emotional link to fear that is aggravating or compromising the person's state of health at this time.

Also, if the area itself is too painful to touch, relief can be achieved by stimulating the meridian at a place further from the actual pain, as this will encourage energy to flow through the entire meridian. The chart in Figure 2 (pg.4) lists some of the meridian associations. These observations were incorporated into the five transformation/element theory, which describes the five qualitative subdivisions of yin and yang. Each of these five phases describes different associations that help to integrate our body processes with the cycles of nature represented by the changing seasons of the year.

Understanding the five transformations allows for observation of the most predominant characteristic energies, which are the source of a person's challenges. Also, revealed are possible interrelationships between the different energy phases.

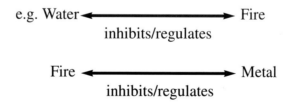

POINTS and TSUBOS

The 360 *points* discovered on the meridian lines were originally referred to as *holes* or doorways to the many channels of energy circulating through the body.

These points serve as storage and generating centers for chi flow (Figure 3, pg.7). From a Western perspective, we could compare these points to batteries and generators situated along an electrical wire or current. Stagnation at any one point prevents energy from flowing freely through the electric wire, causing the total electric charge to suffer. Pain or numbness at these points is a barometer for determining the cause of difficulties. They also serve as effective therapy for alleviation of present imbalances and ideally, for the prevention of pain or dis-ease.

The points were traditionally stimulated through pressure, heat therapy, or by needles. The holes or points, known as *tsubos* (Japanese translation), were given names that described their energetic personalities. For example, the name for Kidney #1 is translated as *"bubbling spring,"* Gallbladder #20 as *"pond of wind,"* and Bladder #52 as *"chamber of spirits."* The names personify the quality of energy inherent to the points. Effective therapy is achieved by stimulating *chi* flow for the associated point being stimulated and by activating those points that best complement the nature of the client and his or her imbalance. An interplay of both experience and intuition are necessary in deciding which points to stimulate.

When *yin/yang, seven chakra, five transformation, meridian,* and *tsubo* theories are integrated with an attitude of compassion and reverence, they provide the basis for a profound system of healing.

As practitioners cultivate health, and are honest about the desire to be of service by supporting other human beings, sessions will be extremely effective. Step by step, the mysteries of healing will be revealed.
"To see the invisible, to touch what cannot be touched." (Wataru Ohashi)

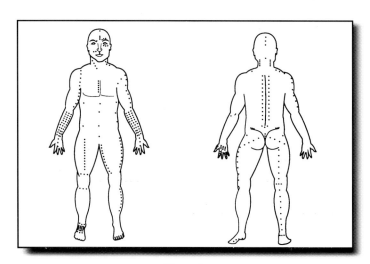

Figure 3

Characteristics of Zen-Touch™

Zen Touch™ is a therapeutic bodywork approach that includes the following concepts:

- Zen Touch™ Practitioners access a deeply relaxed state of mind-body-spirit for themselves and their clients.

- Zen Touch™ Practitioners provide a nurturing, safe, pain-free environment for beneficial body change.

- Zen Touch™ provides benefits for both practitioner and client (i.e., the facilitator feels more flexible, relaxed and rested after each session).

- Zen Touch™ Practitioners utilize deep breathing to facilitate a vital state of being for practitioner and client.

- Zen Touch™ Practitioners develop movements, styles and techniques of their own.

- Zen Touch™ Practitioners follow the momentary needs of the session (i.e., depth of work, tempo and sequence of moves).

- Zen Touch™ Practitioners study traditional Chinese Medicine as a reference standard for Asian Bodywork.

- Zen Touch™ Practitioners experience assessment and therapy with the clients as intuitive discoveries that are based on universal energy dynamics (i.e., the forces of nature as described by Yin/Yang, Empty/Full, the Chakras, the Five Seasons/Transformations, Meridians and Points).

Zen-Touch™ I FOUNDATIONS
BODYWORK PRINCIPLES

Before I outline a possible course of techniques, I would like to suggest five invaluable principles introduced to me at the Shiatsu Education Center of America in New York City, now called the Ohashiatsu Institute. They can be applied to any style of bodywork with great success. They are the fundamental principles applied in Zen-Touch™.

1. Reverence. Always maintain a respect and gratitude for our self, our client and the experience we are sharing together. The ripples of our energetic connection extend infinitely. It is an honor to participate in this sacred communion.

2. Be natural. Project our unique nature into the session. Develop our own style and use only techniques that we are comfortable with. What works for one practitioner/client may be awkward for another. Create a space to facilitate the comfort and well being of both client and practitioner.

3. Be received/avoid pressing. Initially this sounds contradictory, especially since most Asian bodywork incorporates pressure techniques. When the energies of the client and practitioner unite in a meditative or alpha-like state, great regenerative changes take place in the body. This state cannot exist if the practitioner is imposing painful pressing techniques on the client. Rather, if the practitioner allows the weight of his or her body to be received, accepted, and supported by the client, a partnership or unity will be achieved. This oneness initiates a powerful flow of healing energy between the two people.

Listening, in Solitude-Wait...
A path shows itself...
Beckons, pulls me to the ebb of yearning
Now embraced, a wave shudders
Silently smiling

SK

4. Maintain a smooth continuity and flow. Fluidity allows the direction and nature of the session to be led by both client and practitioner. Moving in a continuous flowing manner prevents abrupt insensitive surprise movements that may cause unnecessary tension. Our clients will instead feel completely supported, and this feeling of safety will generate a state of total relaxation in which the conflict of resistance and blockage will freely resolve.

   5. Use both hands. The dispersing quality derived by the use of two hands prevents pain, allowing greater penetration, increased energy movement and maintenance of the relaxed state of the client. Apply the following with a partner (Figure 4): Simply hold a point with your thumb on your partner's forearm and 1) Press with your thumb over one spot while paying attention to his or her pain tolerance; and then, 2) Press two points consecutively along the same muscle. Which technique was painful? Perfection of this balanced technique allows deep penetration while the client remains totally relaxed. (Deep stimulation for some clients is extremely beneficial while others may require lighter stimulation to facilitate benefits.)

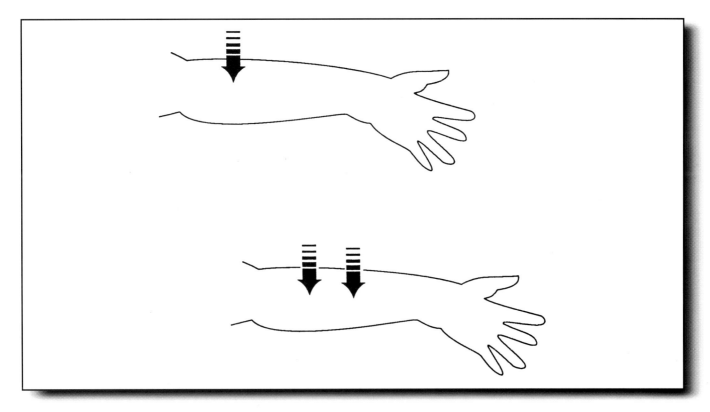

Figure 4

   By integrating these simple methods our bodywork becomes an experience of pleasure. When a gift is given to someone we love - the benefits are mutual.

Selfish am I
To give is to Love
I choose more Love
So give I must

                                   SK

THERAPY and TECHNIQUES

In most styles of Asian massage, the client lies on a soft area on the floor (traditionally on a futon). This floor approach lowers the practitioner's center of gravity, enabling the practitioner to direct the weight from his or her abdominal center toward the client's body. The abdominal center is called the *"Hara"* in Japanese. Moving from the *Hara* establishes a very powerful, balanced, relaxed, energy-generating focus. It prevents arm tension, general fatigue and burnout. The floor technique also frees the knees and feet for use in the session.

Prone Position - The Back and Legs

Step 1

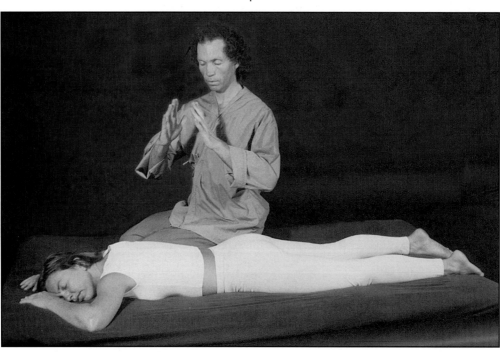

1. Before actually touching the client, take a minute to breathe deeply, center and clear the mind of anything that might get in the way of the session. Create an open space in which the practitioner unites with the client in a beneficially symbiotic energetic flow. Hold the palms in front of the heart center facing each other, move them toward and away from each other until a magnetic vibration is felt. Play with this energetic force and then proceed to extend the palms toward client/partner.

Step 2

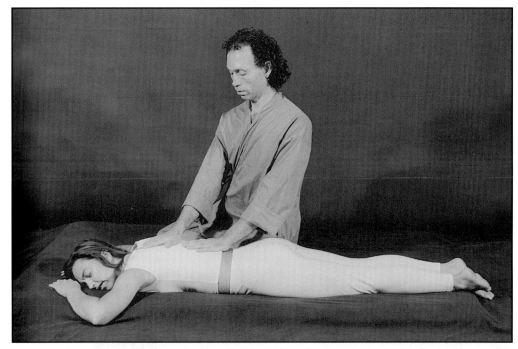

2. Begin by gliding the hands, over the thoracic vertebrae, and continue down toward the lumbar area. This motion serves to introduce the energies of client and practitioner. Is there tightness or flexibility, hot or cold, openness or resistance?

Step 3

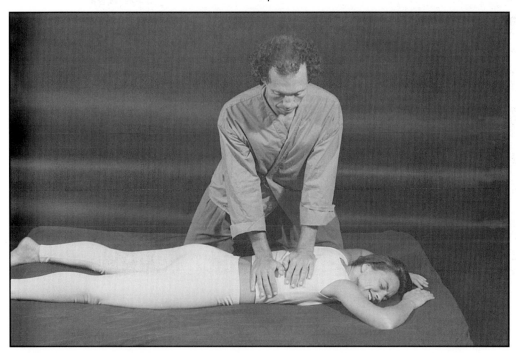

3. Let the client's back support your weight. Sense how much of our weight can be comfortably received. Let the client's back act as a support for your weight. Sense how much weight can be **comfortably accepted by the client.** In a crawling-like fashion, move around the client's body, starting at the upper back and continuing down to the lower legs. In most cases the client will easily support your entire body weight. Feel what it is like to let the client support your weight to the point that if they were not there, you would fall to the floor. Do, however, be careful of the weight on the lower back, knees and calves. Be sensitive. Everyone is different. Make sure the pelvis is tucked under the torso when applying Zen-Touch™. This will maintain straightness through the lumbar vertebrae preventing any lower back strain. This posture actually strengthens any vulnerability in the practitioner's lower back area. Thus, by repeatedly practicing Zen-Touch™, the condition of our lower back becomes more vital.

Step 4

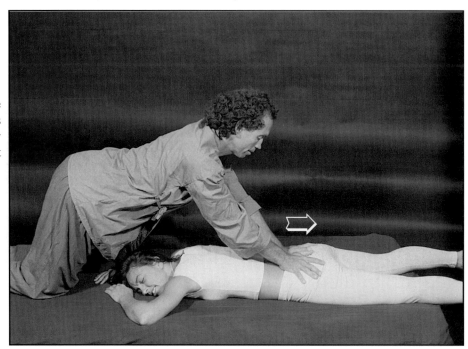

4. While moving around the client's body, begin to sense which areas are tight or loose. Lengthening the body by sending the sacrum towards the feet almost always relieves lower back pain.

Step 5

5. The looser areas often require nurturing, while the tighter areas often require dispersion. For a general technique, keep the palm of one hand stationary on a loose area requiring nurturing (called the *kyo* or empty area), while the thumb of the free hand is moving over and stimulating the tight spots (called *jitsu* or full areas). The stationary palm on the loose areas (called *the mother hand*) accepts the energy that is being dispersed by the moving hand (called the *messenger boy* or *son hand*). To ensure maximum comfortability of the client's lower back it is safest to keep mother hand on the sacrum. Also, **keep mother hand and son hand on same side of the spine.** Listen patiently and feel a vibration under the hands. Breathe deeply and sense the change.

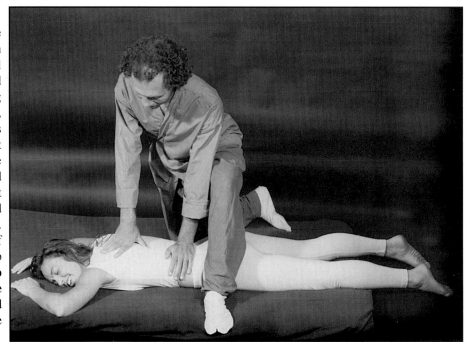

Step 6

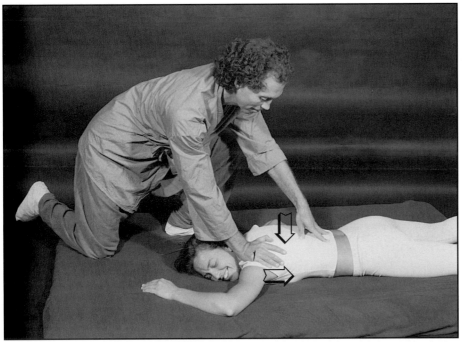

6. In sensitive areas, make sure to use balanced pressure in both palm and thumb hands. Go slowly and gently until the tension releases and the pain subsides. This technique can be applied on any body area, as it initiates great beneficial shifts in energy balancing. It also allows the practitioner to "be shown" the points or tsubos, rather than intellectually deciding beforehand which points to stimulate. Move from the hara. In this position the mother palm hand moves toward the feet while the son thumb moves at a 90-degree angle alongside the spine. Let the palm and thumb be drawn to places that are calling for attention, and let intuition guide the tempo.

Step 7

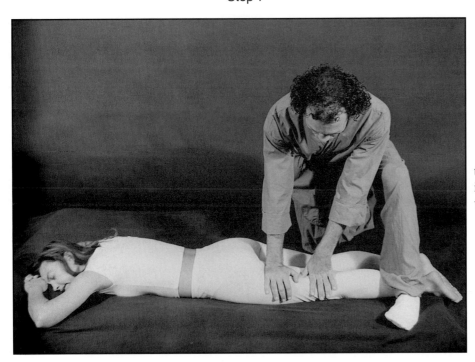

7. Apply the mother/son technique on the back and legs. Son hand initiates the dispersion of energy flow, while mother hand catches or receives it.

In Silent Connection

A quiver? A pulse?

A wave from within

surfaces

Hold, nurture the call

The echoes of life moving toward Balance

Step 8

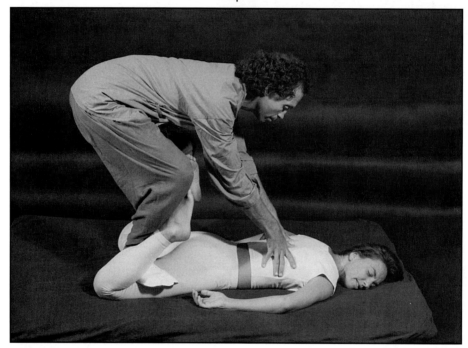

    8. **The Zen-Touch™ Master Technique** — (The appearance of this technique implies great mastery.) Bend partner's knees while standing by their feet. Widen the distance between partner's legs. Step on client's left thigh with the left foot, wrap their foot around the front of the knee to support their lower leg. This allows us to free the left hand and place it on the sacrum. Shift the weight slowly to her left leg while asking if the weight is comfortable. If everything is OK balance the weight on the left side while stepping with the right foot on the client's thigh. Wrap client's right foot around practitioner's knee. Now both hands are free to stimulate points along side the spinal column.

Contra-indications

1)   Pain on the back of thigh — Bladder meridian (which is rare regardless of practitioner's weight).

2)   Tight quadriceps (front of the thigh prevents this stretch) — The "Mini Master" (pg. 15) is usually a comfortable alternative variation.

Step 9

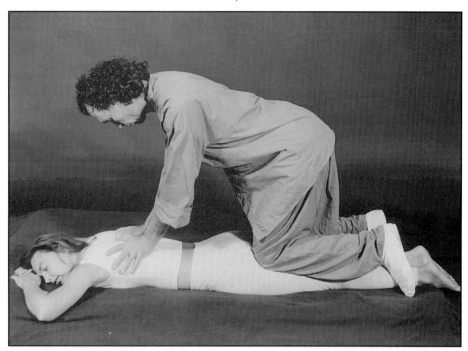

9. **Mini master** — simply crawl on the back of partner's thighs and use palms, thumbs, forearm or elbows on partner's back.

Step 10

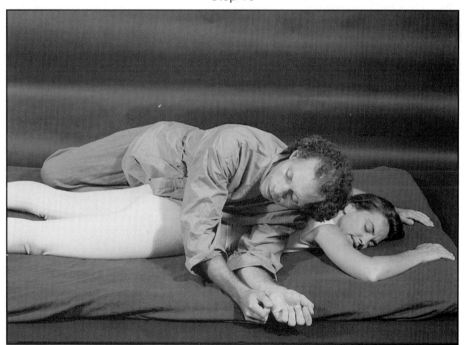

10. **Rolling** — Use palms, forearms and the whole body to gently roll over partner's body. Arch the back slightly over knees and calves to regulate comfortable weight.

Supine Position
Feet, Legs Torso, Neck, Face

Step 11

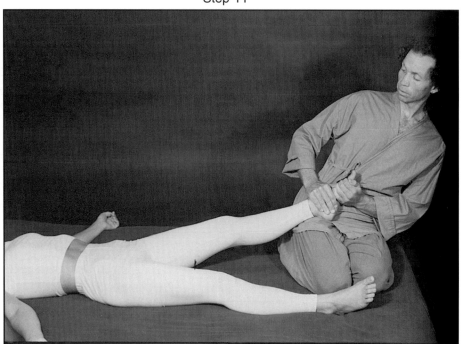

11. Rotating the foot with movement emanating from your Hara (counterclockwise right foot - clockwise left foot). Leaning from the hara opens up the client's whole body. Observe if the client's head moves while you rotate the foot. This signifies we are applying a satisfying rotation. This technique is great for loosening tension in the neck before applying direct touch there.

Step 12

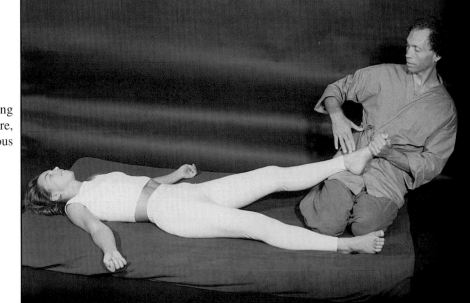

12. Massage the feet using any comfortable technique - pressure, kneading and rotating. Remain conscious of initiating movement from the *hara*.

Step 13

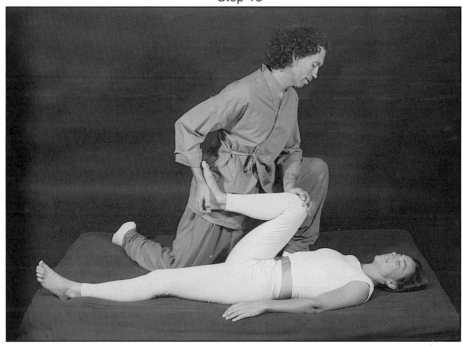

13. **Leg Rotation** — On partner's right leg hold the foot with the right hand and the knee with the left hand. Bend their knee toward the chest and then rotate laterally. Repeat up to 3 times. This rotation opens the hip socket and stretches the leg meridians.

Step 14

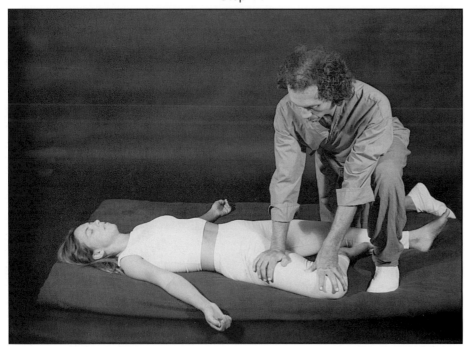

14. Bend client's leg so that the knee falls away from the median of the body. This exposes the meridians on the inside of the leg. (Spleen, Liver and Kidney Meridians). Use the mother/son technique here as well. Use your leg to support your client's knee if necessary.

Step 15

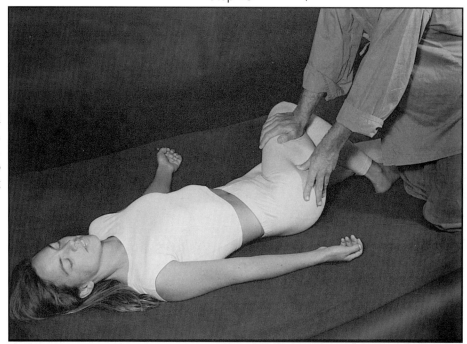

15. The bent leg is then moved toward the median line of the body, where it is supported by the opposite leg. Direct body weight through the palms to stimulate the lateral side of the bent leg (Gallbladder Meridian).

Step 16

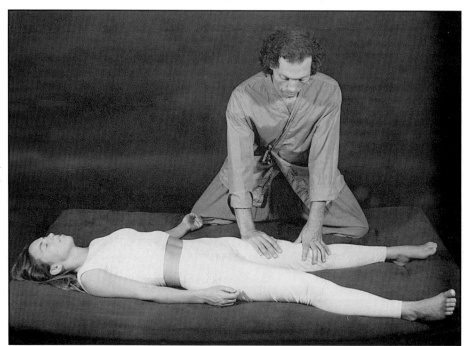

16. Straighten the leg into a parallel position. Stimulate the outside surface of the leg (Stomach Meridian).

Use A and/or B as a transition to other leg.

A

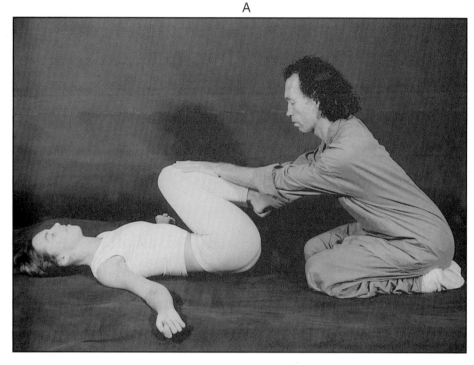

A. Lumber Roll —
Support client's knees with your hands
and circle both ways.

B

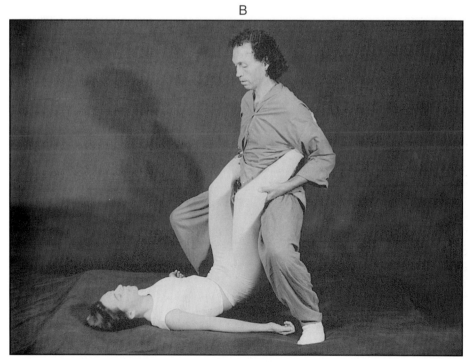

B. Lumber Swing—
Use your legs to lift client off the mat
and swing side to side.

**Repeat steps 11 through 16 on the
opposite leg.**[1]

[1]For beginners a sequence is outlined. Once the practitioner's body is familiar with the moves, I recommend mixing
it up. Improvise where to be and when — it may be redundant to repeat moves equally on both sides.

Step 17

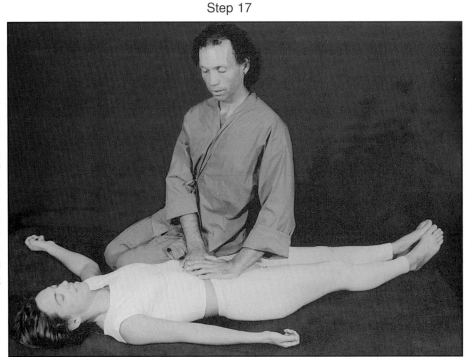

17. While sitting on your knees beside your client (facing their upper torso), use body weight to softly direct the palms into their abdominal area. Keep a stationary mother hand on one area while the moving son hand circles over the abdomen, stimulating all the muscles and organs in the hara area. This is a very effective yet sensitive area to work with. Massaging the hara can reveal the condition of the client and effectively stimulate powerful therapy. Make sure client is openly receiving the weight before going in deep. Be accepted.

Step 18

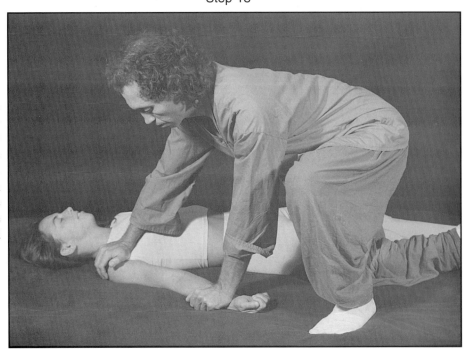

18. Slowly move palms to the client's arm. Extend client's arm away from the torso in 3 positions (steps 18, 19 and 20). Keep a mother hand in the valley where the arm meets the clavicle. Use son hand to move down client's arm in the direction of the fingers. Use the palm of the son hand followed by the thumb to stimulate the anterior and posterior arm.

LUNG/LI meridians on the superior surface of the arm.

Step 19

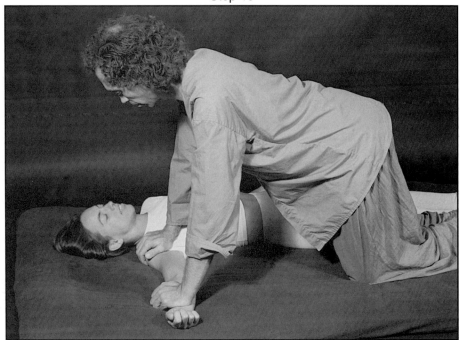

HR/TH meridians on the middle of the arm.

Step 20

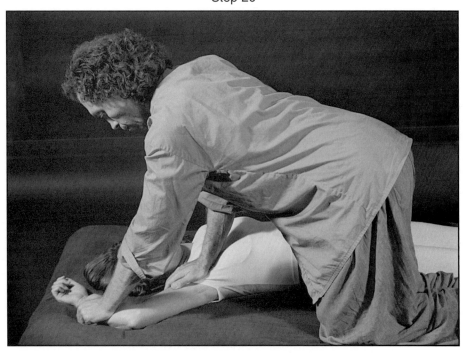

In the bent HT/SI position stimulate both sides on the inferior surface of the arm.

Step 21

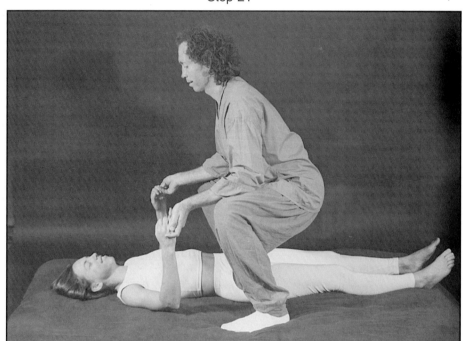

21. Transition to the other arm by holding client's ring and smallest finger. Move your body to freely shake the arms. (This is referred to in class as the *Zen-Touch™ Bougaloo*). When you have *danced* enough, gently lower the arm you have already worked on and repeat steps 18-20 on the other arm.

Step 22

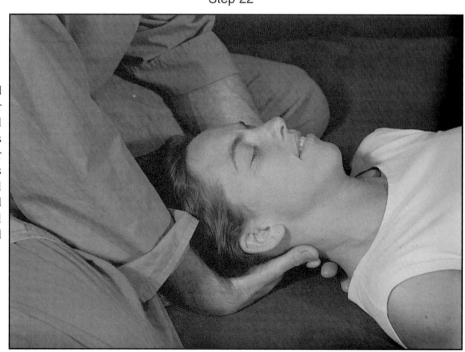

22. **Combing** — Move behind client's head, looking toward his or her feet. Lightly fan hands under the cervical vertebrae one following the other. This is deeply relaxing and serves to move hair away to expose the neck. Keep client's head steadily supported at the occipital ridge with one hand while the other hand gently glides under the cervical vertebrae. Reverse the supporting and moving hands with each stroke.

Step 23

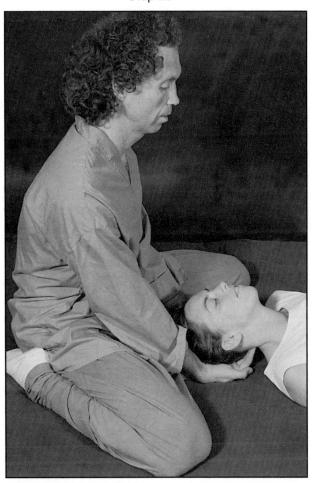

23. **Cervical Rock** — Choose different points alongside the cervical vertebrae to stimulate in an upward direction (90 degrees to the neck). Your client's head will fall back onto your palms. Be drawn in.

Step 24A

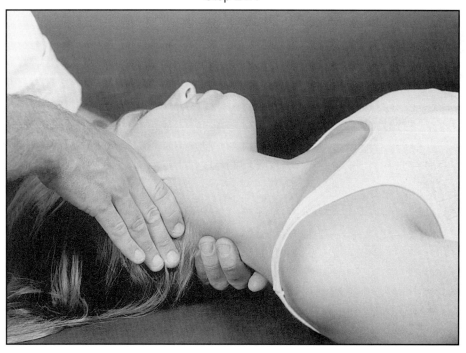

Step 24

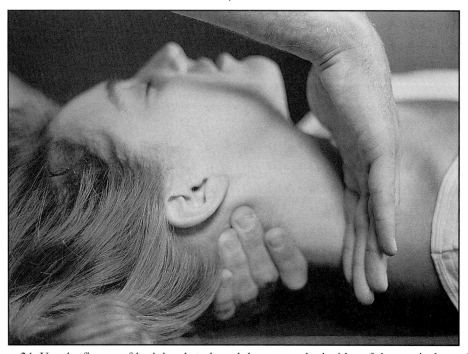

24. Use the fingers of both hands to knead the area on both sides of the cervical vertebrae. Always make sure the head and neck are well supported.

Step 25

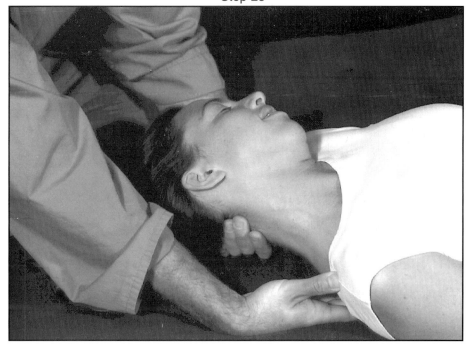

25. **Shoulder Stretch** — Move the head to one side to expose the neck, shoulder and clavicle. Keep client's face in an upward looking position. Begin by moving thumb on a diagonal line from the occipital ridge down to the shoulder. The stationary hand is used to support the head by cupping it under occipital ridge while applying balancing pressure.

Step 26

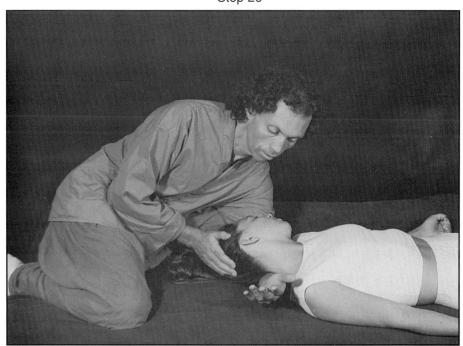

26. **Forearm Roll** — Let client's neck roll along the forearm and apply a gentle downward stretch as the head falls to either side. Repeat with opposite arm.

FACE POINTS

Step 27

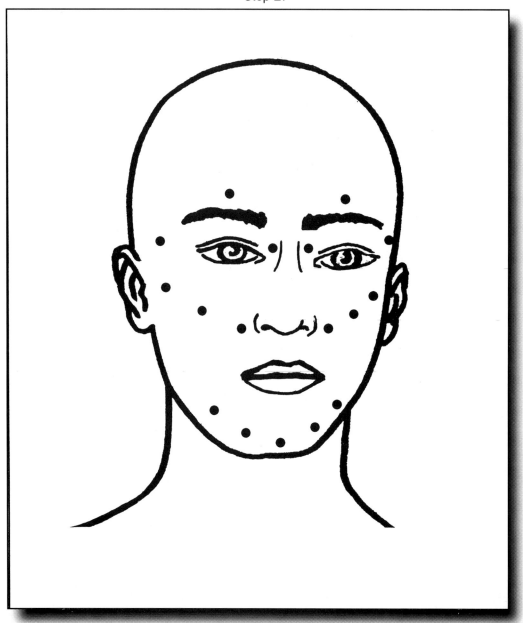

27. Using various fingers, stimulate these points on the face. Use intuition to flow through an effective sequence.

Step 28

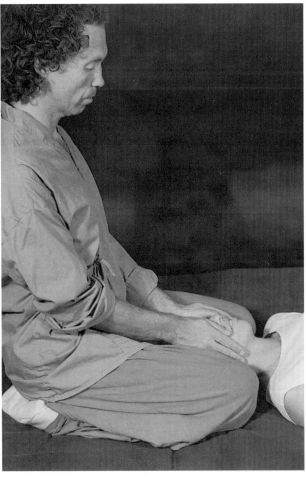

28. End the session by placing palms gently over the eyes. Straighten the spine, breathe deeply, clear the mind, and when ready, slowly remove palms. When the client opens his or her eyes, express "thanks" for being entrusted to share in the mutual experience of communication through touch.

The session I have outlined was influenced by the "Zen" style of Shiatsu as taught by the late Shizuto Masunaga and by the style now called *Ohashiatsu* as taught by one of Masunaga's principal disciples, Wataru Ohashi.

Shizuko Yamamoto facilitates a more vigorous approach to bodywork called *Barefoot Shiatsu* that is extremely effective. Her session incorporates techniques which include walking on the client's back while being supported by a chair, percussion techniques, corrective exercises, and palm healing (energy channeling through the palms without physically touching the client).

The years have shown me that the best technique is the one that works. Apply the techniques and style that best serve you and your clients.

Asian massage offers the body worker a great repertoire of principles to draw from. I encourage practitioners to incorporate the use of body movement initiated from the abdominal center, knowledge of the meridians to stimulate distal areas that connect to troubled places that are too painful to work directly, and use of yin/yang and the five transformation principles to communicate holistically with clients. Most important is the compassion and reverence we bring to our sessions with every client.

Part 2- DEEPER PERSPECTIVES

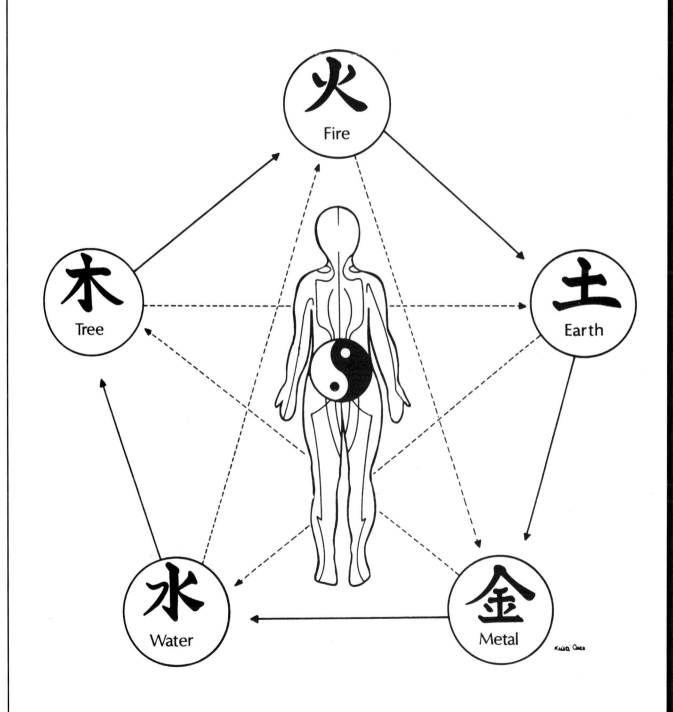

火 Fire

木 Tree

土 Earth

水 Water

金 Metal

YIN and YANG

This Eastern philosophical system demonstrates how the force from heaven called *"yang"* and earth's force called *"yin"* are attracted to each other in a complementary/antagonistic relationship. Observing and comprehending the yin/yang qualities in any phenomena provides a valuable perspective on our inherent drive for balance.

As mentioned previously the growth of plants is a product of sunlight and rain (heaven's downward force), interacting with the soil (earth's upward force).

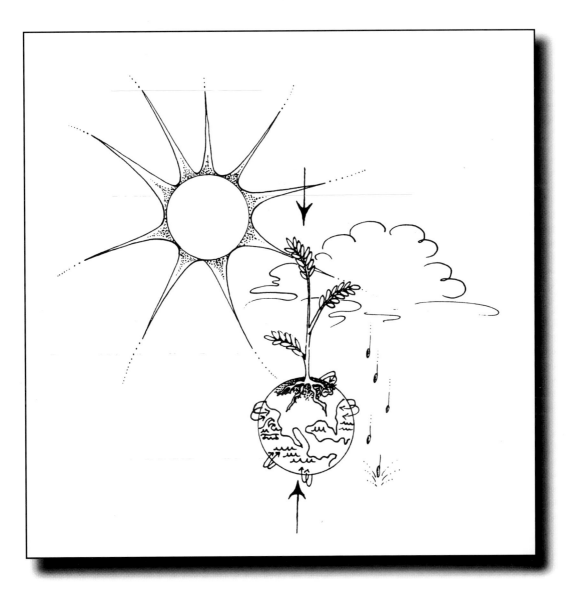

Figure 5

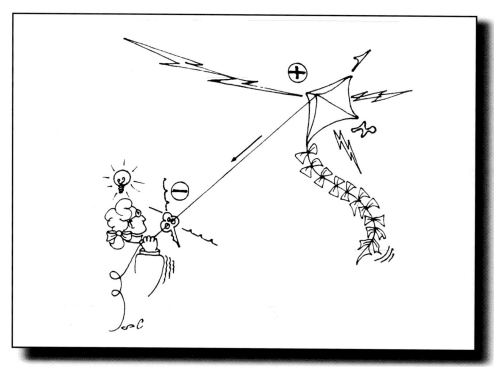

Figure 6

Electricity is produced by the charge of attraction/union between positive
and negative poles.

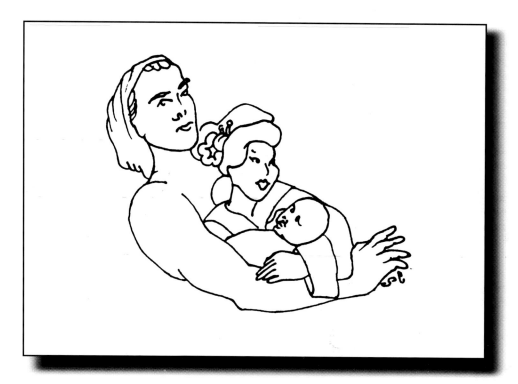

Figure 7

A child results from the relationship between man and woman.

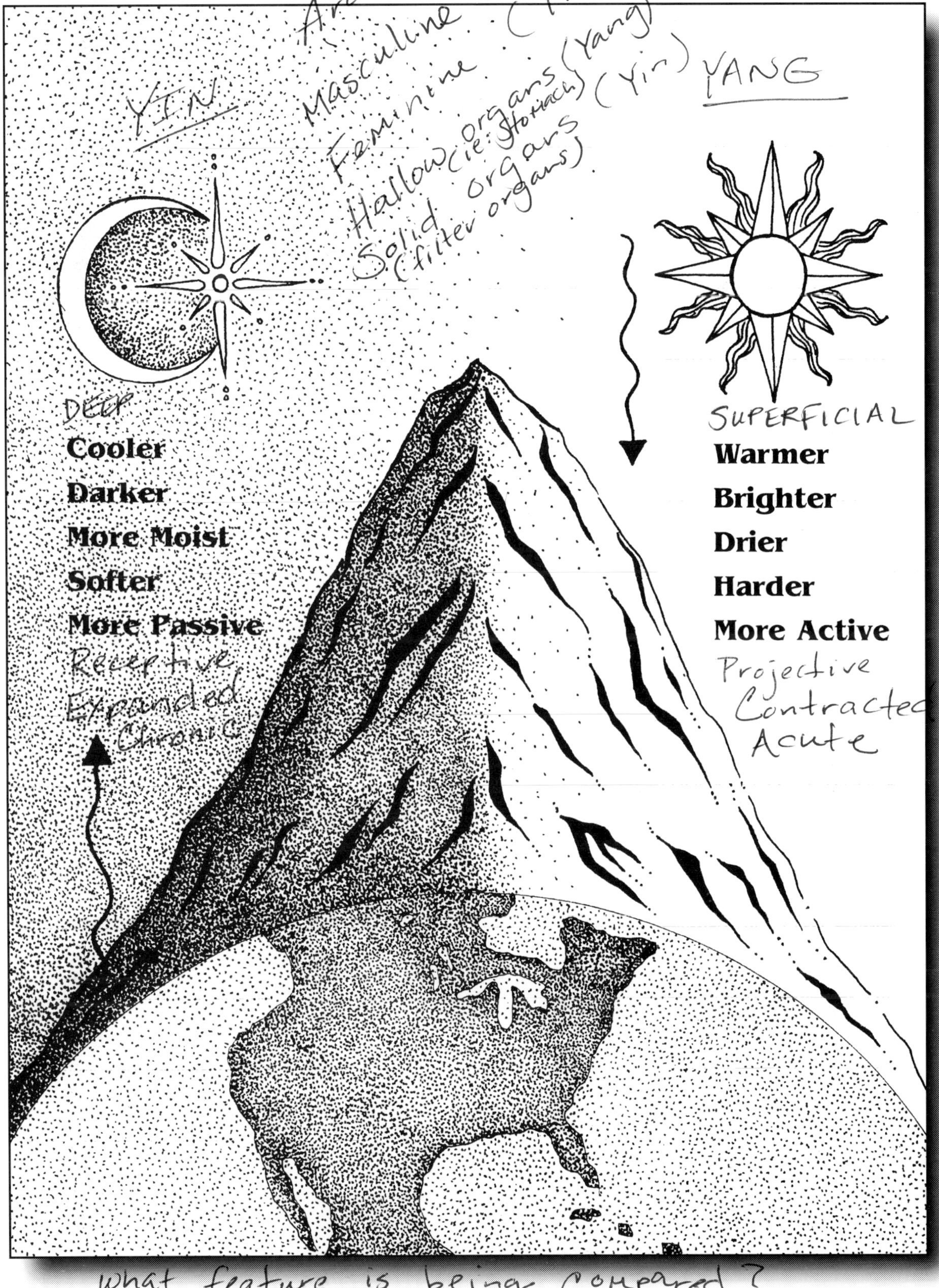

YIN

Cooler
Darker
More Moist
Softer
More Passive

SUPERFICIAL
Warmer
Brighter
Drier
Harder
More Active

Figure 8

The classical Chinese perspective for determining yin or yang was based on the metaphor:
Sunny or Shady Side of the Mountain.

Note that relativity according to daily cyclical changes and the degree of extremes are all influencing determinants of more *yin* or more *yang*. E.g., In a very dry, hot climate the shady side of the mountain may actually show more life activity while the sunny side may be all shriveled/passive.

Yin and *yang* are *relative* descriptions. A rock might be harder than a piece of wood, therefore more *yang*: however, in comparison to a diamond, the hardest of all minerals, the rock is more *yin*.

Also, be careful when comparing the different characteristics of two different phenomena. For instance, which is more *yin*, water or ice? When comparing the two with respect to temperature, ice is colder, therefore more *yin*. When comparing the two with respect to texture, ice is drier therefore more *yang*.

Thus it appears that absolute answers are elusive when classifying *yin* and *yang*. Every phenomenon displays both yin and yang characteristics. If something demonstrates a characteristic that is extremely *yang*, then it also has another equally *yin* characteristic. This dynamic both describes and supports its very existence. For example, if a person displays a very hard, angry outer body expression (aggressive and *yang*) then perhaps inside he or she is housing or protecting an equally soft and vulnerable weakness (*yin*).

George Ohsawa, the father of "Macrobiotics," referred to this paradoxical *yin/yang* dynamic with the phrase "**the bigger the front, the bigger the back.**" In our constantly changing world a certain amount of time might be spent demonstrating an outwardly *yang* expression, while inside, a *yin* expression exists or is building potential, and will eventually surface. The movement derived from balancing *yin* and *yang* describes the extremes that coexist in our ever changing lives.

From a complete or whole perspective beyond time, space, and human emotion, the phrase "out of balance" becomes somewhat misleading. The universe and all its workings are always in balance. It is the parameters or extremes of that balance and their qualitative expressions that account for the differences between phenomena.

For example, a tortoise and a hare are both balanced whole entities, yet their expressions of behavior have very different characteristics. Who is faster? Who is more *yang*? Who won the race? They manifest diverse extremes of *yin/yang* in the balance of their daily lives.

The seasonal nature of such differences will be discussed in the section on the five transformations.

The body has limits as to what extremes it can support and still maintain a somewhat peaceful existence in the physical world. Feelings like fear, love, happiness, sadness, discomfort, pain, anxiety and dis-ease provide signals to guide our journey through life's ever-changing circumstances.

The limits that maintain our survival are like the heights of a see-saw which constantly fluctuate. Movement through extreme parameters is similar to a match that flares up and bums out very quickly. Jimi Hendrix, Jim Morrison, James Dean, Charlie Parker, Kurt Cobain, Janice Joplin come to mind as examples of short-lived intense personalities. Their lives burnt with a passion that could be only briefly sustained. By fine-tuning the parameters of our limits and moderating them, we can more efficiently direct ourselves to achieve long-term goals and dreams.

When our lifespan is represented by a string, it becomes apparent what happens when we live a life of extreme ups and downs. As we moderate lifestyle, lifespan is extended.

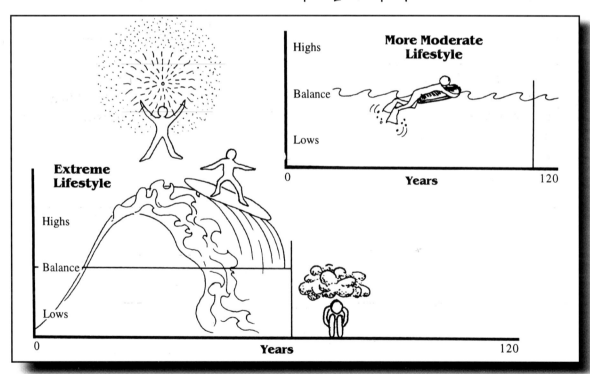

Figure 9

As we work and play at choosing the ranges of fluctuation in the daily balancing of our lives, it is questionable whether we could ever *consistently* experience that place in the middle — "*perfect balance.*" This achievement would produce a state of oneness with the universe and at this point we might be enlightened, disappear, or perhaps be very bored (and therefore imbalanced again).

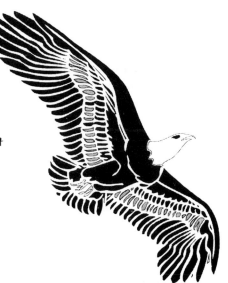

Smiling Intensity
My Fire Burns
Prolonged Ecstasy My Soul Yearns
Moderate my Appetite? Tempered in Concern
Many I know were like shooting stars in the night
Better to burn slow as a candle?
The eagle endures his blissful flight
Or diamond's glittering eternal light
SK

The point of this philosophical discussion on the varying contexts of *yin* and *yang* is that the practical use of this model, when we are working with someone, is complicated, often confusing and impractical to explain.

Traditional Chinese Medicine and ***Macrobiotics***, (a Japanese philosophical life approach) describes **different contexts of Yin and Yang.** *Chinese Medicine* refers to the ***structure*** of earth (*Yin*) as a hard and contracted structure. ***Macrobiotics*** generally refers to the electromagnetic ***force*** emanating from the **earth** (*Yin*). This force moves phenomena in a dispersed and **expanded** direction away from the earth (*Yin*). Chinese Medicine generally refers to the ***structure*** of **heaven** (*Yang*) as ***expanded***. (Just look up on a starry night and you'll see why). Macrobiotics generally refers to the **gravity** *force* **emanating from** *heaven* (*Yang*) as the force that sends mass down to earth...***contracting***. **Both** Traditional Chinese Medicine and Macrobiotics refer to the flow of ***yin*** **meridians** in an **upward moving direction** and of ***yang*** **meridians** in a **downward moving direction**.

Explaining these different *contexts* have been a source of great confusion to students, clients, and professionals. *Lao Tsu,* a Taoist sage, wrote about the illusive/abstract nature of *Yin/Yang*:

The way that can be talked about is not the constant Way.
The name that can be named is not the constant Name.
Non-being is the name of the origin of Heaven and Earth;
Being is the name of the mother of all things.
Therefore:
Constantly in Non-being, one wishes to contemplate its (the Way's) subtlety.
Constantly in Being, one wishes to contemplate its path.
These two come from the same source, but are different in name.
The same source is called Mystery
Mystery and more mystery.
It is the gateway to myriad subtleties.

The following chart lists some of the relative characteristics from which to determine whether phenomena are more *yin* or more *yang*. Note: The frame of reference below relates to the **force** generated from the earth or heaven (as opposed to the structure), and therefore is consistent with the **"forces"** that initiate the meridian direction flow.

Context:	YIN/Earth's (Electro-magnetic force) INITIATES	YANG/Heaven's (Gravity force) INITIATES
Direction of Force:	Toward heaven Centrifugality Expansion/Ascent	Toward earth Centripetality Contraction/Descent
Function of Direction:	Diffusion Dispersion	Fusion Consolidation
Movement Style:	Generally more passive, Slower In <u>Extreme</u>: Ungrounded hyper movement	Generally more active, Faster Focused to earth movement In <u>Extreme</u>: Stuck/Rigid
Temperature:	Colder	Hotter
Light:	Darker	Brighter
Humidity:	More Wet	More Dry
Shape Initiated by Force:	More expansive and loose	More contracted and tight
Texture Created:	Softer	Harder
Atomic Particle:	Electron	Proton
Climatic <u>Effects</u>:	Colder/Contraction	Warmer/Expansion
Gender (See note p. 38):	Feminine	Masculine
Attitude:	More sensitive Flexible, Changeable	More steadfast Solid, Fixed
Work:	More psychological and mental	More physical and social
Consciousness:	More universal, abstract	More earthy, pragmatic
Mental Function:	Dealing more with the future	Dealing more with the past
Culture:	More spiritually oriented	More materially oriented
Dimension:	Space — Spirit**	Time — Soul*

Figure 10

** I define Spirit as the part of consciousness that is cultivated through heartfelt earthly connections and experiences.

* The enriched or developed Soul may provide the essential fuel for the Spirit to express its freedom through infinite dimensions that extend beyond our earthly experiences.

Possible Balance Differences
Between Men and Women

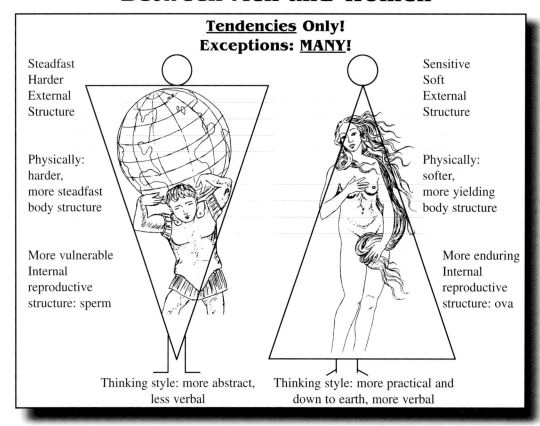

Tendencies Only!
Exceptions: MANY!

Steadfast
Harder
External
Structure

Physically:
harder,
more steadfast
body structure

More vulnerable
Internal
reproductive
structure: sperm

Sensitive
Soft
External
Structure

Physically:
softer,
more yielding
body structure

More enduring
Internal
reproductive
structure: ova

Thinking style: more abstract,
less verbal

Thinking style: more practical and
down to earth, more verbal

Figure 11

GENDER/ATTITUDE

In ancient times men's resilient "yang" outer structure protected them when hunting for food. Their search through unknown territory initiated the development of a more yin or non-verbal intuitive aptitude. Women's more vulnerable, soft "yin" external structure kept them in the villages dedicated to the practical skills of raising children within the community.

Historically, women's external physical vulnerability was perhaps balanced by a practical thinking style with a much greater aptitude for expressing their feelings. Men on the other hand may have a tendency to possess yang (harder) bodies and an equally opposite non-verbal emotional vulnerability. At this late date in time, we are finally realizing that we can mix and match these qualities despite our historical and perhaps biological tendencies.[2]

[2]If the woman/man subject interest you, Seymour's video /audio tapes and his upcoming book *Shaping Our Destiny* contains extended discussion on this subject.

Zen-Touch™ practitioners and instructors use quality-specific words like contracted, expanded, hot, cold, hard, soft, etc. in order to facilitate clear communication with clients who may be confused with the complexities of yin and yang.

Zen-Touch™ also utilizes the expressions "*empty*" (Kyo) and "*full*" (Jitsu). "*Emptiness*" is recognized by the practitioner as a feeling of *wanting* or a *calling out to be held* in a point, meridian, or area that craves attention. "*Fullness*" manifests as a high-energy accumulation calling to be dispersed (e.g. common tension points are found on the top of the shoulders, a "tougher" area that houses tension with more ease than softer, more vulnerable areas like the lower back, abdomen, internal organs, wrists, calves).

Areas where persistent holding and nurturing feel comforting to clients most likely designate an *empty* area. *Empty* areas look and feel like soft valleys and respond with an often-affectionate-like gratitude for attention, usually in the form of holding. If an area is sharply painful, slippery, ticklish, resistant, resembles a high ridge, or feels like a hard mountain peak, then it is most likely *full*, and can be lightly stimulated to disperse its excess energy. The shoulders often demonstrate themselves as *full* areas carrying displaced pain, a signal that ideally motivates people to change. *Full* areas often respond to a more active/dispersing quality of touch in comparison to *empty* areas that usually respond with a slower/nurturing quality of touch.

Zen-Touch™ theory asserts that the original source of any imbalance is *emptiness*: **A feeling or movement in life that has been missing. The body typically displaces the awareness of this source to another area that is perhaps less vulnerable.** For example, when the lower back kidneys/adrenal glands is overworked from drinking coffee the tension is often carried to the shoulders because this area can hold the pain more easily than the more vulnerable lower back.

By initiating a balance between extreme empty and full areas, Zen-Touch™ practitioners directly address the client's greatest imbalance while avoiding the multiple possible classifications of yin and yang.

Zen-Touch™ practitioners also avoid the Japanese words *Kyo/Empty* or *Jitsu/ Full* in an effort to better communicate and educate clients. Instead, Practitioners utilize synonyms which more clearly describe a client's condition (e.g., when feeling a sense of *lethargy* (empty) in the lower back area, therapies to *nourish*, *augment*, and *fortify* the area are initiated and/or recommended).

Sometimes an area will appear full on the surface, but once stimulated, will reveal an underlying emptiness. Simply work the areas as they reveal themselves by nurturing the empty with more holding (usually with the palm) and by dispersing the full with more defined, superficial and (**slightly**) quicker movements (usually with thumb, finger, or elbow). To avoid pain in sensitive areas the following technique can be used (also see Figure 12, pg. 41):

Step 1. Shift weight into the mother hand first.

Step 2. ***Maintain***　this pressure while ***simultaneously***　applying pressure to the thumb of the son hand.

At this point the weight and pressure will be evenly distributed over both hands. If further penetration is welcomed, repeat this procedure layer by layer, remembering to always shift weight and pressure to the mother hand *first,* maintain, and balance with the son hand *second.* (Ask client for feedback, e.g., "How are you feeling? May I go deeper? Is this comfortable?").

This technique disperses sensitivity in the full area, allowing deeper penetration through the layers of the body tissue. This deep penetration, without pain, accomplishes great benefits in energy movement. When applied sensitively, a soothing state of relaxation similar to meditation or dream-like state sleep is experienced. This deep state activates the parasympathetic nervous system and the internal healing/regenerative process.

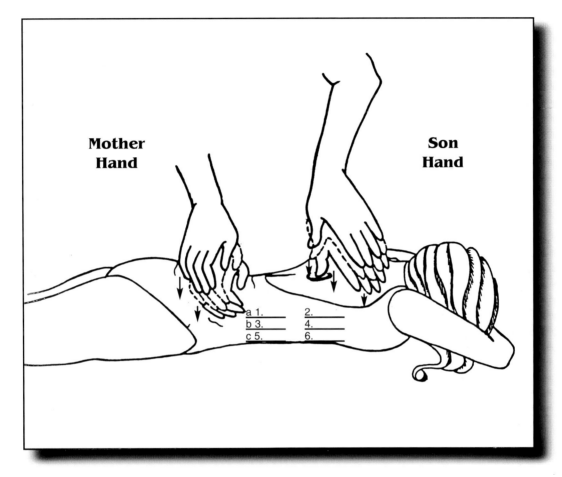

Figure 12

TONIFICATION and SEDATION

The techniques I have just described are often called *"Tonification"* and *"Sedation"*. Empty, deficient areas require filling up or tonification, while full areas require dispersion or sedation.

Quicker movement tends to stimulate the *surface* circulation (e.g., skin turns red affecting the sympathetic nervous system), while slower and consistent pressure tends to affect the *internal* energy flow (parasympathetic nervous system). This internal stimulation is initiated only when pressure is applied *painlessly*.

This procedure creates a sleep-like or meditative state where the surface or outer body remains still and relaxed, while the internal body regenerates. In this internal regenerative state, the peripheral blood circulation slows down (clients often report feeling cold), while the circulation to the *internal* organs is being enhanced. This internal tonification provides energy for activity upon waking.

After fast exercise, like running, aerobics, or swimming, a person may feel temporarily energized immediately after the workout followed by an overwhelming feeling of fatigue and the necessity to recuperate through rest. The same effect is commonly experienced in massage. Generally speaking, techniques done quickly will create a more immediate *surface* stimulation, while slow holding will create a longer lasting *internal* stimulation. The former will usually cause an immediate energy boost, while the latter usually initiates deeper effects, which may manifest several hours later or even the next day. Exceptions depend on the individual's condition. Observe your clients and ask them how they feel immediately after the session and the next day.

A technique I sometimes utilize is to first stimulate the surface with faster percussion, friction, or vibrating techniques followed by holding. This serves to send the surface energy deep into the body and is very effective with deficient energy conditions.

	EMPTY	FULL
Mode of Treatment:		
	1) Tonification (internally)	1) Sedation/Dispersion (externally)
	2) Slow movement or holding	2) Slightly quicker movement
	3) Deeper penetration	3) More superficial penetration
	4) Long term warming effect	4) Long term cooling effect

Figure 13

The body is a myriad of Empty and Full areas. By locating and working the highest Full and the lowest Empty, we will initiate the greatest shift in energy in the least amount of time.

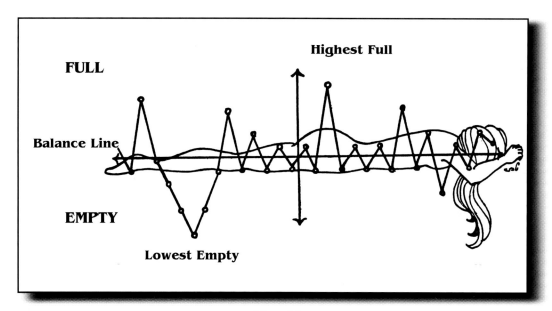

Figure 14

We will be doing less, yet facilitating more. The concept of Empty and Full is the first step in learning to work on someone with a minimum of analytical thought. Eventually we will find ourselves in a clear, or *"no mind"* state, intuitively moving in and out of different areas.

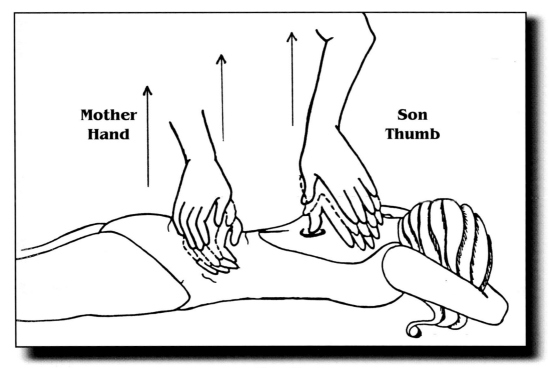

Figure 15

Point Impressions

This technique characteristic of Zen-Touch™ has facilitated wonderful results with many people:

1) Hold a point for an extended period of time (at least 2 minutes) while breathing very, very slowly.[1] Remember to keep the connection between mother and son hands.

2) Move the body very slightly allowing the client to inhale, yet always maintain pressure and energetic contact. Great surges of energy moving through the meridian system between mother and son hand are commonly felt when the connection between both hands is balanced.

3) To exit the point, the practitioner moves his body away as slowly as possible while exhaling. As it may take 2 or 3 minutes to fully disconnect, maintain an energetic connection and slight pressure on each inhale and always move away while exhaling. (See figure 15)

The impression of the point will remain with the client for a long time. If done on several points, the client's body will feel a continued stimulation regardless of where you are presently working.

---

[1]Holding points or areas for a long time 5, 10, 15, 20... minutes generates very deep changes. Great sensitivity to the receptivity of the client is required with this method as the body releases and balances deeply held emotional memories.

THE CHAKRAS

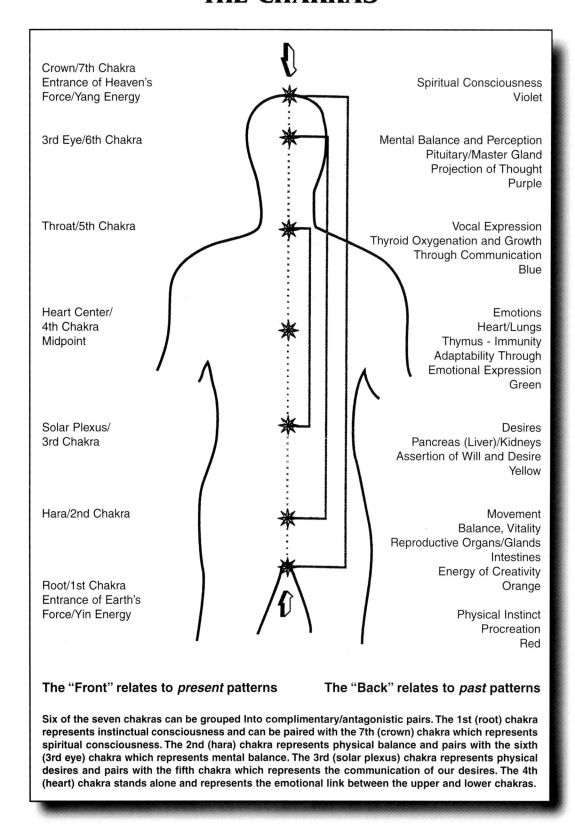

Crown/7th Chakra
Entrance of Heaven's
Force/Yang Energy

Spiritual Consciousness
Violet

3rd Eye/6th Chakra

Mental Balance and Perception
Pituitary/Master Gland
Projection of Thought
Purple

Throat/5th Chakra

Vocal Expression
Thyroid Oxygenation and Growth
Through Communication
Blue

Heart Center/
4th Chakra
Midpoint

Emotions
Heart/Lungs
Thymus - Immunity
Adaptability Through
Emotional Expression
Green

Solar Plexus/
3rd Chakra

Desires
Pancreas (Liver)/Kidneys
Assertion of Will and Desire
Yellow

Hara/2nd Chakra

Movement
Balance, Vitality
Reproductive Organs/Glands
Intestines
Energy of Creativity
Orange

Root/1st Chakra
Entrance of Earth's
Force/Yin Energy

Physical Instinct
Procreation
Red

The "Front" relates to *present* patterns　　　The "Back" relates to *past* patterns

Six of the seven chakras can be grouped into complimentary/antagonistic pairs. The 1st (root) chakra represents instinctual consciousness and can be paired with the 7th (crown) chakra which represents spiritual consciousness. The 2nd (hara) chakra represents physical balance and pairs with the sixth (3rd eye) chakra which represents mental balance. The 3rd (solar plexus) chakra represents physical desires and pairs with the fifth chakra which represents the communication of our desires. The 4th (heart) chakra stands alone and represents the emotional link between the upper and lower chakras.

Figure 16

THE CHAKRAS

The "Chakras" are seven major centers that lie along the body's central energetic core (also referred to as the primary channel). From the crown of the head to the groin area, these centers are the source of vibration and energy for all body mechanisms. Please refer to the diagrams in Figures 16 and 19 (pg. 46 and pg. 50).

The **first** or **"root" Chakra** serves as *the "entrance" point of earth's upward electromagnetic force*. This Chakra represents the root of our physical instinctual consciousness, e.g., our automatic sexual, procreation, and survival responses and drives.

The **seventh,** or **"crown" Chakra** serves as *the "entrance" point of heaven's gravity downward force*. This Chakra represents the root of our universal consciousness, e.g., spiritual understanding, and intuitive ability to respond to our spiritual path.

Heaven's force and **earth's force** are attracted to each other. They seek each other along the primary channel, collide and express themselves at the remaining five Chakra centers. At each of these five places, characteristics of our ever-changing condition are revealed and effected.

Our **second,** or **"hara" Chakra** *facilitates physical movement/balance, creative vitality and action, and plays a great role in influencing our elimination and reproductive functions*. This area is also known as the reservoir of *"Chi"* (life force energy). As our reservoir fills with vital energy, the over flow circulates into the higher centers.

The **third**, or **"solar plexus" Chakra**, *facilitates our "desires"; our "hunger for life."* It directly influences our stomach, pancreas, spleen, liver, and gallbladder functions.

Note: The *umbilical cord* navel (our original connection with mother's nurturing) lying between the 2nd and 3rd Chakra centers suggests why these areas of our physical vitality and balance (2nd chakra) and our desires (3rd Chakra) are so deeply effected by ties to closely connected relationships. Cultural, racial, familial ties and any personal interactions that initiate great inspiration or frustration may catalyze deep energy shifts that affect the functions of organs located here. Ideally we take benefit from the power provided by feelings. The lower position for these Chakras tends to stimulate physical body manifestations that are less consciously associated with our emotions or philosophical and spiritual responses. E.g., An imbalance here may manifest as lower intestinal or reproductive difficulty (2nd chakra) or blood sugar imbalances (3rd chakra — pancreas or liver related) without a clear awareness of the emotional/philosophical or spiritual pattern connected to the physical difficulty. Imbalances in the higher Chakras demonstrate more obvious connections between behavioral conditions and physical imbalances, e.g., "stress" induced headaches.

The **fourth**, or **"heart" Chakra**, *facilitates our emotional expression and directly influences heart and lung functions.* Its position (midpoint on the primary channel), determines its natural role as the bridge between our physical and spiritual experiences. So often, people feel frustration, anger, or sadness because their heart Chakra's function of linking grounded daily living experiences (lower Chakras) with spiritual consciousness (upper Chakras) is compromised.

The **fifth**, or **"throat" Chakra**, *facilitates communication.* The grounded source of our willpower and life desires originate in the lower Chakras while our ability to *express* our path finds outlet here.

The sixth or **"third eye" Chakra**, *facilitates mental balance and foresight.* Our five senses are directed through the powers of the mind to maintain balance between thoughts and action. The tendency to *over* analyze often shows up as tension between the eyebrows.

As we move toward "Health, Happiness and Harmony," we experience a greater sense of freedom in our lives. As we clear the primary channel and cultivate the charge in these energetic centers, we will clearly see and feel the *unity* of physical and spiritual balance.

As an assessment tool, the Chakras can be very helpful. It is commonly believed all body structures and organs originate from the vibrations created by heaven's and earth's force colliding at each of the Chakras. Thus, if we observe stagnation at the different Chakra centers, we can initiate change by working complementary meridians to create balance. For example, the posture of a person whose upper body (particularly the head) reaches forward suggests heightened activity in the *upper* Chakras. The person may be experiencing mental pressure which creates tension and pain in the neck and shoulders. A possible therapy could be to stimulate the meridians in the legs to initiate activation of the *lower* Chakras.

The Chakras can be worked directly in sitting, standing, supine or prone positions. Also, *"palm healing"*, a technique where the palms are placed over the different Chakras at a distance from the body, can also be employed. Here, the practitioner is working more with the body's projected energy field, instead of a more direct stimulation to the meridians through the body tissue. I find working the back relates to a person's connection with past patterns, while working on the front relates to his or her present relationship with the future.

Figure 17

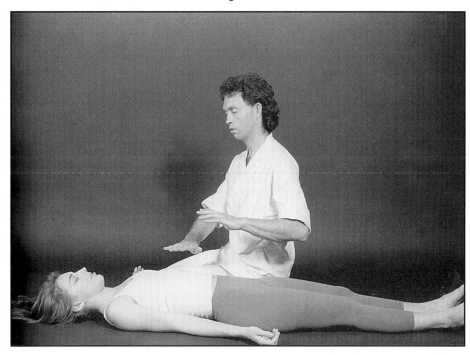

Figure 17
One traditional technique includes
chanting various sounds while palm
healing in order to increase the
vibrational field. For example, the
"aaah" sound stimulates the lower
Chakras. The "oooh" sound stimulates
the middle Chakras and the "mmm"
sound stimulates the higher Chakras.
Thus, we have the popular chanting
phrase a-u-m."

Figure 18

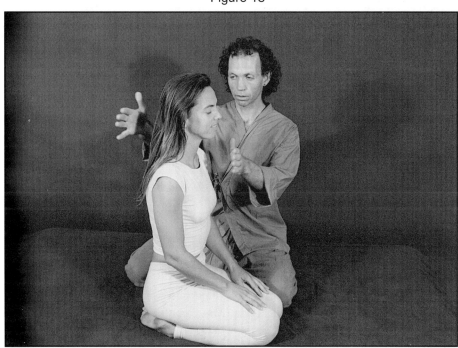

Figure 18
Move your hands toward and away from
each of the chakras. Which draws you in
most? Does one send you away?
Describe the quality or feeling...Draw it.
Allow yourself to perceive relevant
phrases, colors, images...

A Suggestion to Connect – A Silent Bridge
Volcanic Relief
Satiates A Yearning Chasm

CHAKRA BALANCING

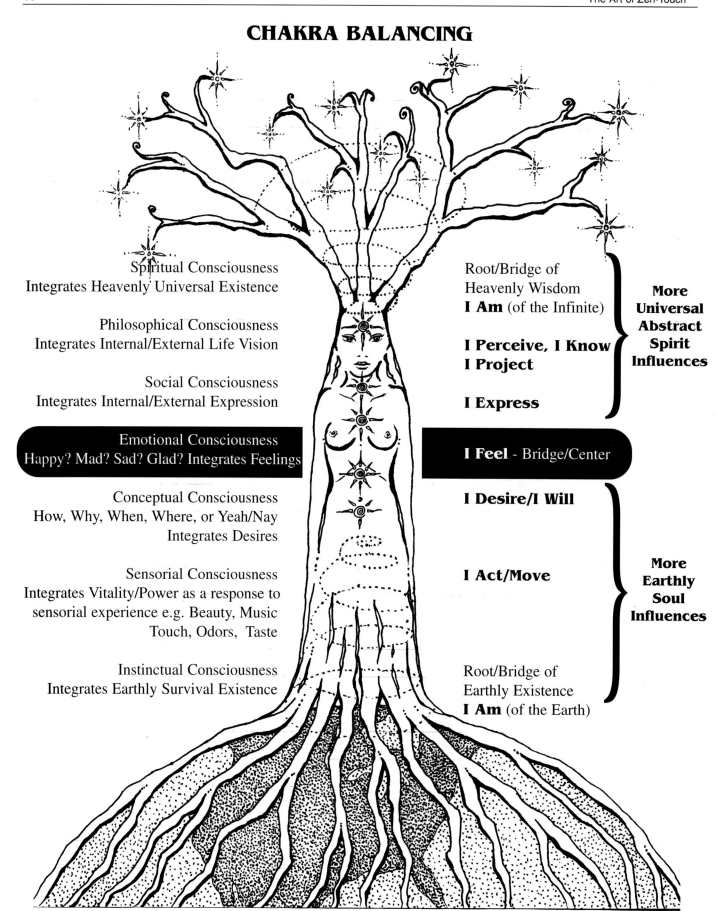

Spiritual Consciousness
Integrates Heavenly Universal Existence

Philosophical Consciousness
Integrates Internal/External Life Vision

Social Consciousness
Integrates Internal/External Expression

Emotional Consciousness
Happy? Mad? Sad? Glad? Integrates Feelings

Conceptual Consciousness
How, Why, When, Where, or Yeah/Nay
Integrates Desires

Sensorial Consciousness
Integrates Vitality/Power as a response to
sensorial experience e.g. Beauty, Music
Touch, Odors, Taste

Instinctual Consciousness
Integrates Earthly Survival Existence

Root/Bridge of
Heavenly Wisdom
I Am (of the Infinite)

**I Perceive, I Know
I Project**

I Express

I Feel - Bridge/Center

I Desire/I Will

I Act/Move

Root/Bridge of
Earthly Existence
I Am (of the Earth)

**More
Universal
Abstract
Spirit
Influences**

**More
Earthly
Soul
Influences**

Figure 19

Both Ancient Traditions and Quantum Physics contend that energy is the fundamental component underlying all phenomena. To effect the body at this fundamental source can create powerful changes.

The concept of Empty and Full directs us to the primal source of a body's imbalance. As we detect and effect the Area, Chakra, Meridian, or Point that is most Empty and that which is most Full, our connection with this individual's pattern of imbalance will be very profound.

Initiating change toward balance through these energy extremes creates ripples of vibration which effect all our bodily experiences - e.g., pains, immune responses, emotions, mental or spiritual limitations, tensions, accumulations, etc.

When the Empty and Full pattern is mobilized, clients often find their own answers. They ask questions about diet, exercise, and lifestyle that surprise the most experienced practitioner. They heal themselves.

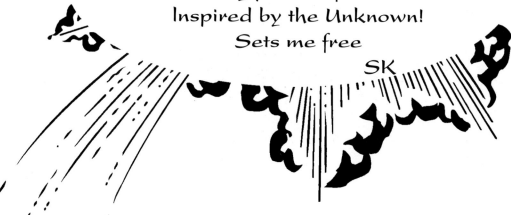

Years of Stuckness
difficult yet predictable
fear of change! Safety in the Known
stale as it may be

One day a Spark,
Who knows from where it came
The vision of New Beauty adorns me
My path Unfolds
Inspired by the Unknown!
Sets me free

SK

THE FIVE TRANSFORMATIONS

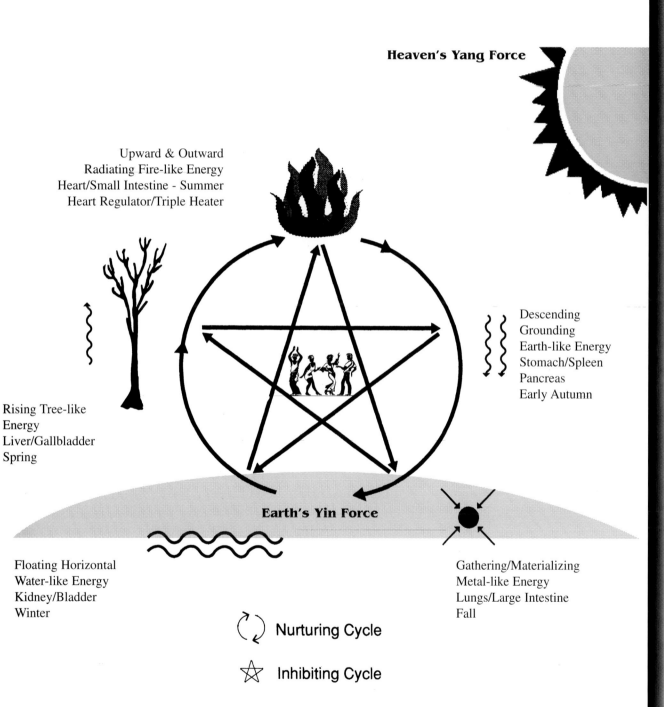

Heaven's Yang Force

Upward & Outward
Radiating Fire-like Energy
Heart/Small Intestine - Summer
Heart Regulator/Triple Heater

Descending
Grounding
Earth-like Energy
Stomach/Spleen
Pancreas
Early Autumn

Rising Tree-like
Energy
Liver/Gallbladder
Spring

Earth's Yin Force

Floating Horizontal
Water-like Energy
Kidney/Bladder
Winter

Gathering/Materializing
Metal-like Energy
Lungs/Large Intestine
Fall

Nurturing Cycle

Inhibiting Cycle

The Five Transformations

Every phenomenon demonstrates a unique, qualitative balance between *yin* and *yang* characteristics. To better understand the nature of life, the five transformations theory was introduced. It helps us to observe how *yin* and *yang* interact with each other within a system of cyclical change that parallels the seasons of the year.

This model describes how the cycle of floating, rising, radiating, descending, and gathering, constantly changes and repeats its movement quality throughout the hours, days, seasons, and years of our lives. Each phase contains different characteristics of *yin* and *yang*. These five transformations assist us in our perception of the different *qualitative* aspects of *yin* and *yang*, as opposed to measuring only their *quantitative* values.

For example, while summer and winter both manifest characteristics of *yin* and *yang*, their qualitative expressions are more unique than the sum of their individual measurable differences.

The concept to embrace here is how the nature of the different energy movements and transformations effect different people throughout their daily lives.

As we view the seasons with their characteristic movements, we will discover which movements are lacking in a person's life and which may be overemphasized.

Note: The common term 5 "elements" is a great over-simplification of this "energetic" system. The use of words like Water, Wood/Tree, Fire, Earth, and Metal are mere examples of the descriptions: Floating, Rising, Radiating, Descending/Grounding, Gathering/Completing.

(≈) **Water-like energy flows.** It is similar to sleep or hibernation, where energy regenerates and potential is cultivated like a seed, dormant underground, awaiting spring. This floating energy represents the behavior pattern described by the well-known phrase "going with the flow."

If the free expression of this energy is blocked, a person might experience caution, fear, or even paranoia when confronted with too great a change. We could compare it to the feeling of being suddenly awakened from a deep sleep. Disorientation, a rush of adrenaline, and a shocking scare, are possible adverse reactions experienced when an extreme stagnation of our floating energy is influencing our personality. When flowing freely, water-like energy expresses itself by motivating a person to courageously flow from one change to the next, appreciating the challenges and growth that their difficulties stimulate. Just as water flows to assume the shape of any container or boundary, so too, will a person flow to accommodate any situation. "Boldly going where no one has been before." (*Star Trek,* Gene Rodenberry.)

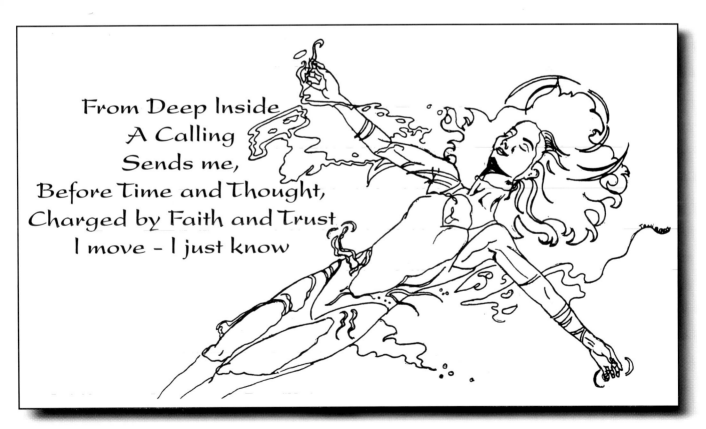

From Deep Inside
A Calling
Sends me,
Before Time and Thought,
Charged by Faith and Trust
I move - I just know

Figure 20

(⟨♨⟩) **Rising, tree-like energy** can be compared to the spontaneous upward movement of a seed sprouting through the earth to catch the brightness of the sun's rays. Spring is here! Spontaneity, creativity, organization, drive, and patience, are all expressions of free moving, rising tree energy. When stagnated, the enthusiasm of this bursting quality may express itself as indecisiveness, frustration, and anger. Control is also a key word here. Anger is either turned inward to maintain an air of being "in control," or rises, thus expressing itself in a "loss of control" through shouting or violence.

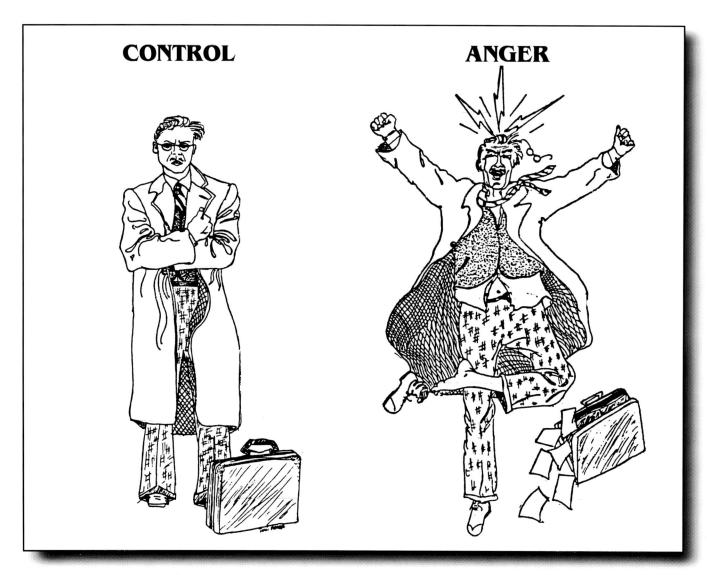

Figure 21

Spring freshness caresses every pore
Meet it. I must.
Catch the Sun
Awakening, Rising – I REACH...Yes!
SK

(☿) **Fire-like upward and outward energy** represents the flourishing and radiant inspiration of life. Summer excitement. Rising tree energy creates the idea that sparks fire-like energy into full bloom. Fires can burn with great excitement, and they always require fuel. Stagnation in this phase might be expressed as hyperactivity, extreme mood swings ("flaming" ups and "burnt out" downs), and a desire for stimulation from others to fuel the flame. (e.g., laughter and applause). A person manifesting balanced fire energy expresses himself as a consistent and peaceful charismatic source of light to which others are charismatically attracted.

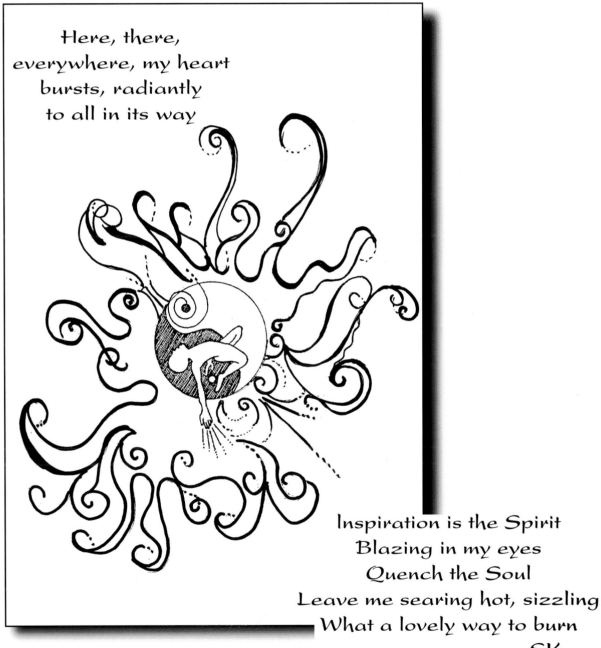

Here, there, everywhere, my heart bursts, radiantly to all in its way

Inspiration is the Spirit
Blazing in my eyes
Quench the Soul
Leave me searing hot, sizzling
What a lovely way to burn
SK

Figure 22

(🌏) **Descending soil-like energy** takes the inspiration of fire phase and starts grounding or carrying through in movement toward manifestation. Resources and energy are necessary to accomplish tasks. If a person's energy is too slow, heavy, or inconsistent, he will seek support. In extreme cases, pity or martyrdom may be tools which a person uses to draw in people as his lack of stamina and resources prevent him from confidently carrying through ideas by himself.

On the other hand, understanding the importance of others can initiate great compassion in a person's free expression of soil/earth energy. This energy transformation represents the mother-earth image, where nurturing oneself overflows in generosity to connect with and serve others.

Listening, Embracing
Love
The warm touch raptured in safety
Focus to endure
Sweetness so pure
SK

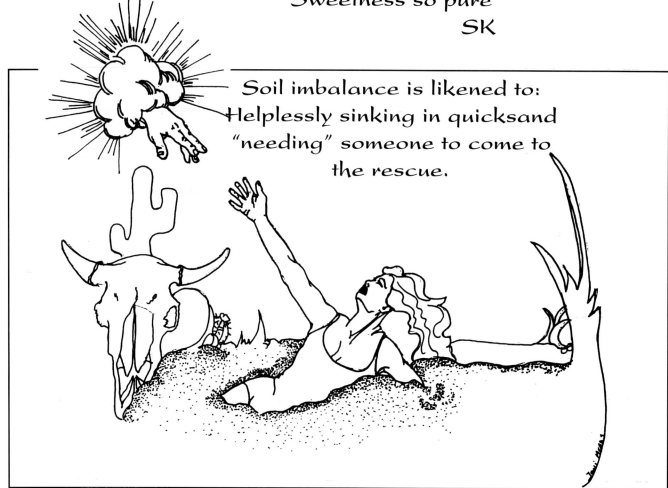

Soil imbalance is likened to: Helplessly sinking in quicksand "needing" someone to come to the rescue.

Figure 23

(→🌀←) **Gathering metal-like energy.** This final energetic phase represents completion and achievement of personal goals - the finished product. Individuality, commitment, devotion, determination, independence and material success are all possible characteristics of this phase, as are stubbornness, rigidity, guilt, feelings of being stuck, difficulties with trust issues, and isolation.

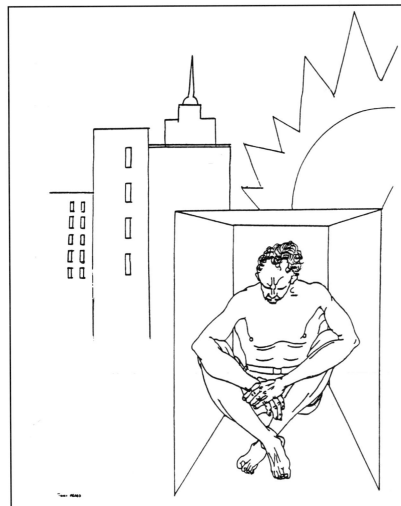

Ah .. Tis me - Finally
"I" defined
Just in Time
Keep this Knowing - can It be Forever?
Alas life changes
Stay the same? - Moulting, Shedding skin
Metamorphis, Uniquely blending
Ah .. Tis still ME

SK

Figure 24

LIFE CORRESPONDENCES OF
THE FIVE TRANSFORMATIONS OF ENERGY

Movement:	Flowing	Rising	Radiating	Grounding	Gathering
Elemental Example:	Water	Tree	Fire	Soil	Metal
Parallel Organs:	Kidney, Bladder	Liver, Gallbladder, Heart Regulator, Triple Heater	Heart, Small Intestine	Stomach, Spleen/Pancreas	Lungs, Large Intestine
Emanating:	Openness, Courage, Flow	Direction, Freshness, Spontaneity	Excitement, Variety	Nurturing, Safety, Compassion	Dependability, Regularity
Natural Ability:	Flexibility, Adaptability	Creating New Activity	Expansion and Inspiration	Focus, Carry Through	Completing, Moving On
Natural Difficulty:	Integrating change, "flow"	Loss of Freedom	Focusing on One Endeavor	Being Alone	Spontaneity, New Ways
Extreme Reaction:	Fear, Insecurity, Backing Away	Anger when Controlled, Frustration, Impatience, Rage	Excitement, Laughing, Scattered, Manic ups and downs	Pity, Suspicion Gossip, Victim, Blames **others**, "Abandoned"	Sadness, Guilt, Depression, Blames **self**, Controlling, Inferiority, Shame
Free Expression:	Adventurous, Adaptable, "Flow"	Spontaneity, Organization, Patience, "Fresh"	Radiant and Inspiring, "Charismatic"	Empathetic, "Supporting"	Dependable, Successful, "Complete"
Relationship Aptitude:	Seeing Overall, Big View, Intuitive, Awareness	Discovering, Empowering, New Direction	Inspiring, Passionate	Bonding, Listening	Commitment, Devotion
Relationship Drawback:	Easily Detached	Power Quest	Multiple Interests	Insecure, Blaming Others	Guilt, Shame, Being Right or Wrong
Emotive Body Response:	Shivers	Gripping	Hyperactive, Nervous	Sobbing, Energy Draining	Stuck, Isolated Barren
Voice:	Apologetic, Groaning, Timid	Directing, Shouting	Excited, Verbose	Singing, Whine	Monotone, Choked
Natural Direction:	North	East	South	Center	West
Activating Environment:	Cold	Wind	Heat	Moisture	Dryness
Harmonizing time of day:	Night	Morning	Noon	Early Afternoon	Sunset
Harmonizing Season:	Winter	Spring	Summer	Early Fall	Autumn

Figure 25

Continued

Movement:	Flowing	Rising	Radiating	Grounding	Gathering
Moon Cycle:	New Moon	Half Increasing	Full	Waning Full	Half Decreasing
Physical Association:	Bones	Muscle, Tendons, Ligaments	Blood Vessels	Interstitial Fluid, Lymph	Skin
Physical Branches:	Head Hair	Nails	Face Color, Complexion	Breast, Upper Lip	Breath, Body Hair
Physical Fluids:	Urine	Tears	Perspiration	Saliva	Mucus, Snivel
Sense:	Hearing	Vision	Taste	Touch	Smell
Harmonizing Taste:	Salty	Sour	Bitter	Sweet	Pungent
Identifying Imbalanced Odor:[1]	Putrefying e.g., Urine	Oily, Greasy e.g., Rancid Oil	Burning, Scorched e.g., Burnt Toast	Stale Sweetness e.g., Old Perfume	Rancid e.g., Fecal Matter
Complexion Hue:	Grayish	Dark Brown, Yellow, Green	Red	Orangish, Yellow	Sallow, Pale White
Facial Indicator:	Ears, Below Eyes	Eyes, Between Eyebrows	Tongue, Tip Nose, Cheeks	Mouth, Nose Bridge	Nostrils, Cheeks, Lower Lip
Harmonizing Grain:	Buckwheat, Beans	Barley, Wheat, Rye	Corn, Amaranth, Quinoa	Millet	Rice
Harmonizing Vegetables:	Seaweeds (cooked), Beans	Rising Greens, e.g., leeks, green onions, celery, sprouts	Large Leafy Greens, e.g., kale, collards, dandelion	Round Vegetables e.g., squash, pumpkin, cabbage, cauliflower	Contracted Plants, Roots, e.g., radish, onion, burdock, carrot
Beneficial Fruits:[2]	Winter and Dried Fruits	Spring Fruits	Summer Fruits	Late Summer Fruits	Autumn Fruits
Harmonizing Color:	Dark Shades; blue, purple, black	Bright, Fresh; green	Intense; fluorescents, red	Soothing Rustic; yellow, orange	Pure; white
Harmonizing Recommendations:	Small Challenges	Free Play and Recreation, Avoid Pressure, e.g., Competition	Focus, One Step at a Time	Supportive Environment Accept Role as "Participant"	Variety Forgive

Figure 25a

Classifying a person's health difficulties within the above associations provides insight into the specifics that ideally reveal the source of his or her imbalance, e.g., if a person revealed cold in the bones, hearing problems, a dark complexion, frequent urination and a timid attitude, it would be obvious that their kidneys required attention. Abdominal and back assessment could reveal whether this energy network was empty or full. Extreme life situations are more easily detected. Less obvious scenarios require a deeper intuitive connection.

[1] Ideally, your experience of these smells will be subtle. In extreme cases they are somewhat difficult to endure.
[2] Indigenous to various climatic/geographic areas.

PHYSIOLOGY OF THE ORGANS

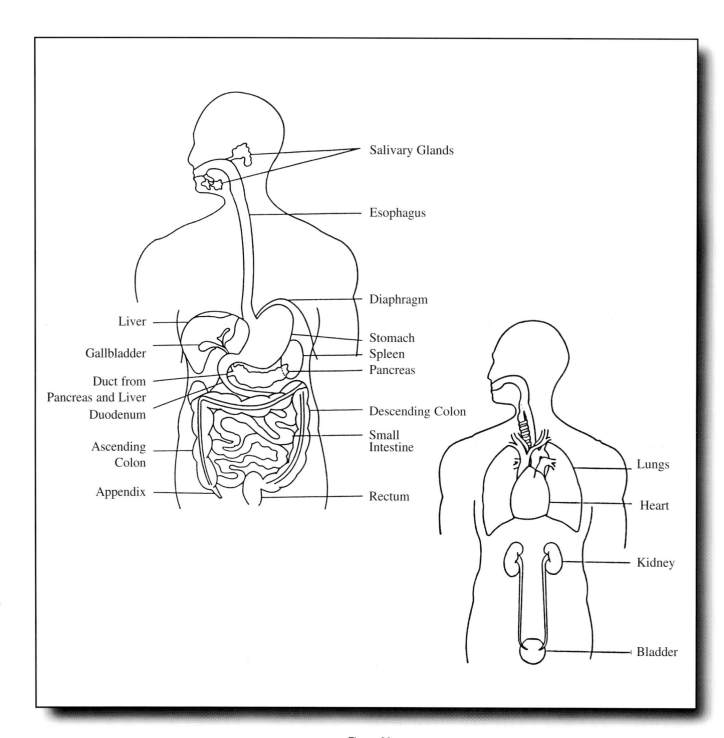

Figure 26

PHYSIOLOGY OF THE ORGANS

Element	Physiology of the Organs	Five Transformation Correlation
Floating WATER	**KIDNEY** - Filtering of blood, maintains mineral balance. **BLADDER** - Elimination of waste through urination.	Keeps the blood, our internal ocean Clear and Energized, thus providing the brain with Clear, Adaptable Thinking. Mineral balance conducts electricity/charge of courage.
Rising TREE	**LIVER** - Liver produces bile to aid in digestion (fats especially) and stores bile in gallbladder. Detoxifies toxic substances, e.g., drugs and inhalants. Maintains blood-sugar level with the pancreas. Metabolization, biotransformation of proteins, fats, carbohydrates and toxins. The liver performs over five hundred and eighty-nine bodily functions. **GALLBLADDER** - Distributes the secretions produced by the liver.	Spontaneously Directs our Dreams into Action. Likes to <u>direct</u> with speed accuracy and freshness - <u>the opposite of</u> **Metal's Logical Control** which actually inhibits **Liver's Love for Dynamic Movement.**
Radiating FIRE	**HEART** - Circulation of the blood. **SMALL INTESTINE** - The majority of the yet-to-be-digested foods are assimilated here.	Circulation and Assimilation of Life's Inspirations. Surging, Expressing Charismatically.
Grounding EARTH	**STOMACH** - Gastric acid, enzymes, and mucus - breaks down food, empties in one to four hours. **SPLEEN** - Production of white blood cells - breaks down red blood cells, mineral storage. **PANCREAS** - Production of insulin and glucagon which balances blood sugar for energy. Pancreatic enzymes aid in digesting major nutrients (i.e., carbohydrates, fats, proteins).	Provides resources and reserves to Carry Through, Focus and Nourish our Life Appetites.
Gathering METAL	**LUNGS** - Gather oxygen and expel carbon dioxide. **LARGE INTESTINE** - Storage and absorption of water and vitamins and elimination of waste. (Appendix— Lymphocytes which aids in immunization produced here.)	The independence of self is initiated with our first breath as we leave the womb. Upon completion of our goals we are impelled to let go, and enter the flow again to deepen our life experience.

We all experience different physical, psychological, and spiritual manifestations of these five energies at different times in our lives. If a person remains in one phase for too long, a situation of extremes might arise. A typical example would be the person who, after accomplishing a task successfully (metal/gathering energy), fails to see the importance of moving on to the next challenge (water/flowing energy), and consequently, feels depressed or stuck. They may experience "physical and mental constipation." As we integrate our personal lives with the constantly changing environment we intuitively shift from one phase to another efficiently flowing through any and all circumstances.

While we experience the various transformation energies at different times in our lives, it is particularly interesting to observe how one or two phases might dominate the nature of a person's character. For example, some people "float" through their life circumstances (water-like energy), while others spontaneously shift from one situation to the next with great speed and spontaneous direction (rising energy). Some people explode with flamboyance and unpredictability (radiating fire-like energy), while others naturally attract supportive people and relationships to themselves (nurturing soil-like energy). Gathering, metal-like, energy motivates people to move through their life cycles with a consistent logical, dependable motion. Observe peoples' most common or rare behavior patterns. This may be a clue to their most full/excess and empty/deficient life movements.

Nurturing and Inhibiting Cycles

Referring back to page 53, we find that as we move in a clockwise direction, each phase nourishes the next. Water nourishes/generates trees, tree nourishes/ generates fire, fire nourishes/generates soil, soil nourishes/generates metal, and metal nourishes/generates water.

The following is an example of the *"nurturing cycle"*:

If we sleep well (floating phase), we are able to rise easily (tree-like/rising energy) and **spark** our creative powers to flourish (fire-like radiating energy). Our inspiration motivates the **grounding** of ideas. Focusing our resources (earth-like descending energy) is necessary to bring our plans **down to earth** and will promote the **completion** (gathering/metal phase) of our activities. Our ability to manifest (metal-like/gathering energy) imparts the confidence to follow deeper dreams (water-like flowing energy).

Looking inside the circle on page 53, we find that water regulates/inhibits fire, tree regulates/inhibits soil, fire regulates/inhibits metal, and metal regulates/inhibits tree.

The following is an example of the *"inhibiting cycle"*:

If we lay around sleeping all day, it would be impossible to create inspiration in our lives (water inhibiting fire), or too *many* inspiring ideas may prevent us from completing one important task (fire inhibiting metal).

The nurturing and inhibiting cycles describe two of the many movement/ element relationships.

Any phenomenon or activity that imparts qualities inherent to one of the Five Movements (e.g., people, personalities, behavior, food, or exercise) can impart these same qualities to the person who partakes in them. For example, root vegetables like carrots or burdock root with their more downward focused, metal-like energy affect people differently than spices, like cayenne pepper, which evoke an expansive, radiating, fire-like energy.

Such applications combined with nourishing/inhibiting influences, and all the associated characteristics listed in Figure 25 (pg. 60 and 61), provide us with a detailed, complex system to work with. Valuable as it is, I find this kind of knowledge once understood, is best left dormant, as the analytical approach more often than not, gets in the way of an effective session. The knowledge (when understood) will surface when we require it.

For example, if a person wears red, behaves with hyperactive emotional mood swings, complains of pain in their left arm, and likes hot peppers, one might logically assume that working their fire energy — heart and small intestine — is the best place to focus on in the session. Perhaps sedating their rising energy (liver/ gallbladder) would provide less nourishment for their active fire energy?? Tonifying water energy (kidney/bladder) might initiate better results by inhibiting (dousing) their fire energy??

I have found that my best confirmations of the five transformations showed themselves independent of any premeditated or conscious application of their theory, only to find out, after a successful session, that a correlation to the five phases could be made. For example, in the situation of a client who was experiencing a flush complexion, neck pains, headache and a slight fever, instead of working those areas directly, one look at his feet just drew me in. I found an incredible *Empty* feeling in Kidney 1 point *"bubbling spring"* at the ball of the foot. Rather than analyze that magnetic attraction, I felt it was more important to just be there and stimulate the area. In retrospect, after the therapy, it was easy to see how nourishing water energy at Kidney 1 could control his excess heat and upward radiating energy.

At some point, we put our knowledge on the back burner and simply place our hands on the area of the body that is calling out to be touched. The next step is feeling the quality of touch that stimulates these areas most efficiently — soft and light or firm and penetrating? A gathered, focused, and "pinpointed" quality or perhaps a floating wave-like and tender approach? We eventually develop what Wataru Ohashi calls a *"skinship"* with our client, i.e., an intimacy of touch communication. This is the place from which great healing is initiated.

Buried in lessons and logic
Mind searches
This or That?
Where is the Truth?
Slip away,...Silence Surrenders...
Ahah!
SK

THE MERIDIANS and POINTS

The meridians are vessels of energy that flow throughout the body. Because the word meridian literally means *"imaginary line"*, many professionals prefer the word *"channel"*. These energy conductors circulate our internal life force, which regulates all the body's metabolic functions. The flow of this energy affects us physically, emotionally, and spiritually.

There are 12 major meridians, which are described in a system of pairs that correspond to one of the five transformations. Each pair consists of a *yin meridian*, which originates from earth's upward yin force, as well as a *yang meridian*, which originates from heaven's downward yang force. For example the pair associated with water-flowing energy consists of the Kidney/Bladder meridians. The Kidney meridian (*yin*) begins at the ball of the foot and moves upward into the chest. The Bladder meridian (*yang*) begins in the head, continues down, alongside the spine and ends in the little toe.

Although the meridians are sometimes described as one-dimensional lines, which begin and end at various points, they are more metaphorically imaged as an interwoven web of continuously connected flowing energy that circulates vitality throughout every aspect of the human essence.

The following illustrations depict the *external* or most surface meridian pathway shown on *one side* of their *bilateral* locations. The *internal* channels of each meridian are shown in some of the recommended reading references listed at the end of this text.

The Yin Meridian Lines

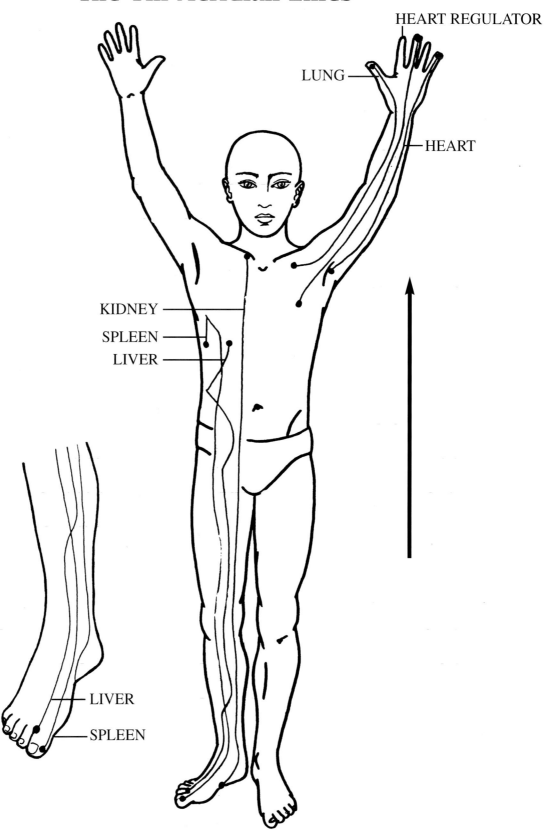

Figure 27

The Yang Meridian Lines

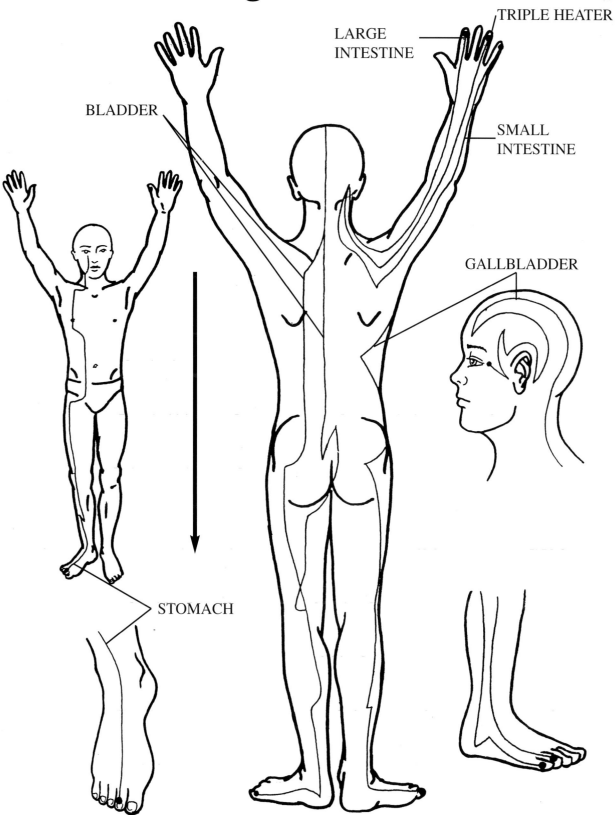

BLADDER

LARGE
INTESTINE

TRIPLE HEATER

SMALL
INTESTINE

GALLBLADDER

STOMACH

Figure 28

The inner "infinity-like" line shows the meridians according to the "Chinese Time Clock" which asserts the specific time of day that "Chi" moves through each meridian. See Footnote on figure 29.

Chinese Time Clock

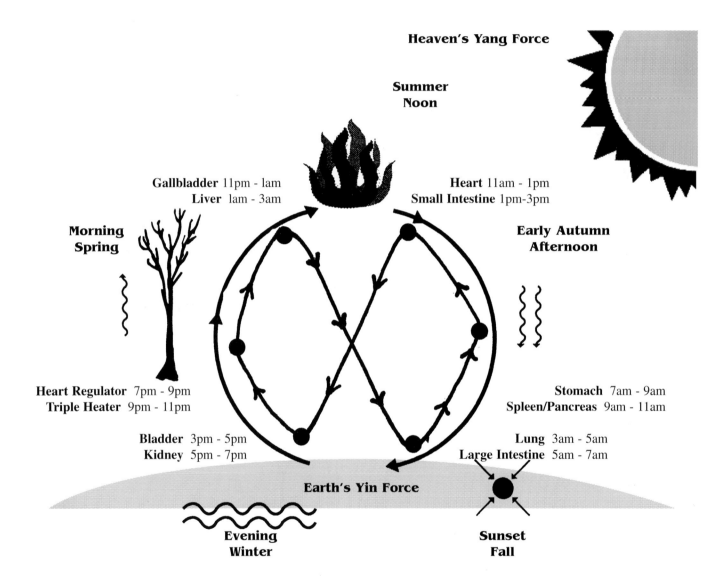

Figure 29

Energy also moves very obviously through the meridians corresponding to the times of day and season. When assessing or applying therapy in correspondence to these three possibilities consider them all. E.g., Asthma in the evening could be a LU, KI or winter association. I have personally experienced more accurate clues of one's condition according to the time of day (morning-liver, noon-heart, etc.) and with seasonal indications compared to the Chinese clock associations. I always consider all three.

HOLES / POINTS / TSUBOS

Along the meridians lie access points or holes which the Japanese call *"tsubos."* These points act as reservoirs or generating centers for the meridians' energy. Each point has been found to affect a number of different body functions. When stimulating these points, the practitioner will feel a quality of fullness or emptiness. Zen-Touch™ maintains that the best effects are achieved when the points find us, rather than when we spend time analytically searching for them.

The use of "touch" is very different from stimulation by a needle. Points, meridians, and areas that will potentially create change through touch will call out to our hands for attention. These places, which magnetically draw us in, are the most powerful catalysts of change. If our palms and thumbs feel comfortable and well received, then we are truly initiating beneficial changes. I encourage the development of this sense rather than pondering with a book about which of the documented 360 points <u>should</u> be stimulated to obtain a result. Experience demonstrates that there are actually an infinite number of points awaiting discovery.

On the other hand, I do recommend sitting down with a detailed and thorough book to study the traditional points. In more acute symptomatic applications knowledge of the different points and their experiential effects may prove very useful. Also, the often-metaphorical names of the points provide insight to the deep philosophy this system originates from. Familiarity with tradition may open our intuition to the myriad of possible applications for use with a wide range of people.

The following are some illustrations of the meridians and major points, which have repeatedly proven to be very effective initiators of energy movement in my work. Reflect on the physical and energetic functions of each meridian to perceive how stimulation at the various points can effect the indication listed.

It is possible that a point on kidney, heart, stomach or any other meridian would be helpful if it was the meridian source most closely involved in the individual's condition. The listed indications for therapy are most effective when the specific meridian of the chosen point is the predominant source of imbalance. For example, while Lung #1-Center of Gathering-includes "asthma" as an indication for therapy, it may be just as likely to alleviate "asthma" by stimulating any of the other meridians depending on the individual's unique life circumstances.

Note: The 12 major meridians flow bilaterally (i.e., on both sides of the body); the diagrams presented show them on one side.

LUNG MERIDIAN

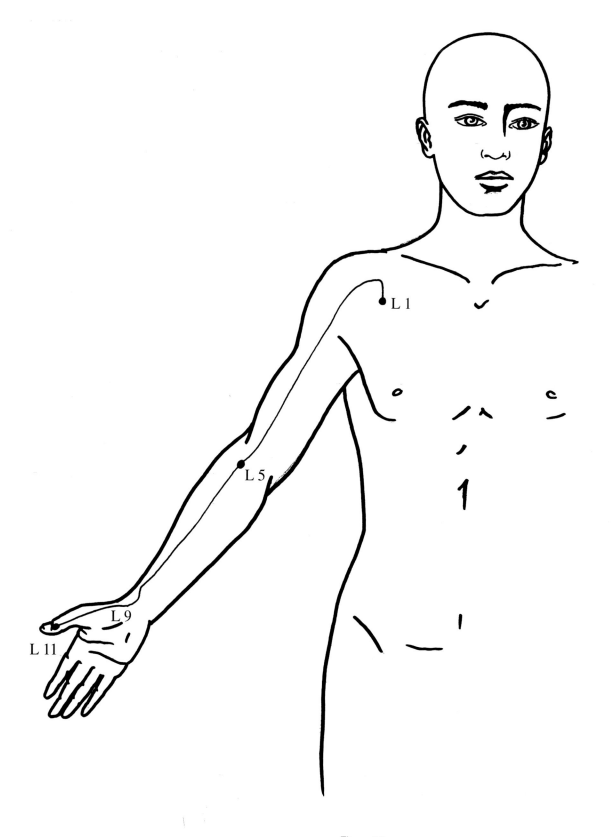

Figure 30

LUNG MERIDIAN (Yin)

At birth we take our first breath independently of our mother. The umbilical cord is severed and we are for the first time in nine months breathing on our own. Physical exchange of gases, O^2 in and CO^2 out also parallel the exchange/communication with our physical *and* social environment. Communication with others establishes *self*-understanding and influences the energy flow through this meridian, as does letting go and forgiveness of the past. The lungs represent the gathering of energy from our environment for the purpose of establishing wholeness and individuality. The lungs also represent our first layer of protection from extremes in our external environment. A common initial entrance for emotional and physical *dis-ease* is through the lungs. Breathe!

Looking at You
What do I see
Turbulence or Trust
Breathing Two Different Sides of Me

Lung #1 - Chu Fu (Center of Gathering) - between the 1st and 2nd ribs in the valley formed where the clavicle meets the shoulder.

Therapy for: This point and the surrounding area are very effective for colds, coughs, asthma, and any lung connected problems.

Lung #5 - Shoku Ta Ku (Indentation in the Stream) - in the cubital crease on the outside (radial side of the tendon). Bend your elbow to find the crease.

Therapy for: Elbow problems, breathing difficulties.

Lung # 9 - Tui En (Great Stagnation) - in the depression on the radial side of the radial artery below the wrist.

Therapy for: Unconsciousness revival, sore throat, and overall balancing point for lungs.

LARGE INTESTINE MERIDIAN

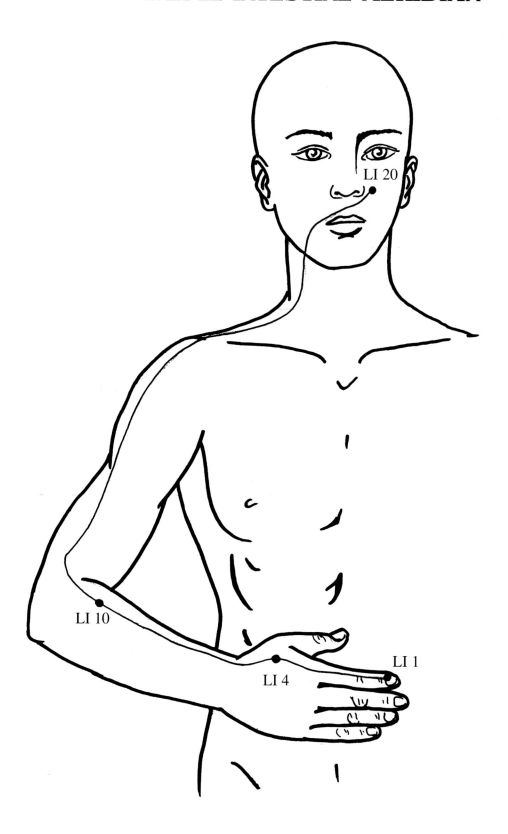

Figure 31

LARGE INTESTINE MERIDIAN (Yang)

The LI meridian with its absorption and elimination functions acts as a barometer for how well we are completing and eliminating the fuel of our daily lives. Our fuel comes from food, air, and also includes the energy provided by all our social interactions. Constipation, diarrhea, and all intestinal symptoms reflect challenges related to environmental integration. Also, productivity and efficiency of manifesting creative expression is often influenced by how well we have eliminated patterns of stagnation from the past.

Events of the past...resentment?
Do I still hold?
Spirit come forth
Reabsorb, Forgive
Gratitude for the lesson
Move on.
My greatest choice calls . . . Truth . . . Destiny . . . NOW.
SK

LI #1 - Sho Yo (Yang Merchant) - at the base of the nail on the thumb side of the index finger.

Therapy for: Fever and diarrhea.

LI #4 - Go Ko Ku (Meeting Mountains) - in the mound between the index finger and the thumb, just under the 2nd metacarpal bone. Make a fist, and the formed protrusion marks the point.

Therapy for: Toothache, headache, hic-cough, diarrhea, skin rash, general health.

LI #10 - Te San Ri (Three Miles) - 1 1/2 inches below the crease in the bent elbow.

Therapy for: General health point, arm fatigue, toxin release.

LI #20 - Gei Ko (Welcome Smell) - in the small grooves in the side of each nostril.

Therapy for: Sinus trouble, facial tension.

STOMACH MERIDIAN

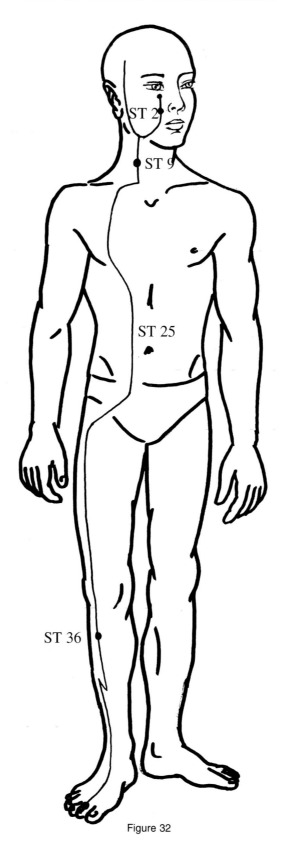

Figure 32

STOMACH MERIDIAN (Yang)

The stomach represents our appetite and hunger for life. Our designs, desires, and the tempo we choose to pursue them at, are all reflected in the condition of the stomach network.

In Writing?
Words?
Action?
A Song?
Desire persists, time motivates.
My Focus Strong
SK

ST #2 - Shi Haku (Four White) - below the eyes in the depression set under the cheekbone.

Therapy for: Facial paralysis, headache, sinus troubles, toothache.

ST #9- Jin Gei (Welcome Human) - about 1/2 to 2 inches from the middle of the larynx.

Therapy for: Hypertension, throat problems, asthma.

ST #25 - Ten Su (Center of Borderline) - two cun* lateral to the navel.

Therapy for: Intestinal problems, abdominal pain, insomnia.

ST #36 - Ashi San Ri (Three Miles) - 3 cun below the knee cap on the lateral side of the tibia.

Therapy for: General health point (especially for men), tired legs, preparation for change of season.

*Note: The term *"cun"* (pronounced "tsoon") is the Chinese measurement, which denotes the approximate distance represented by client's 2nd phalange of the middle finger (the area between the first and second knuckle). For example, the pupil of an eye is 1 -1½ cun away from the bridge of the nose.

SPLEEN / PANCREAS MERIDIAN

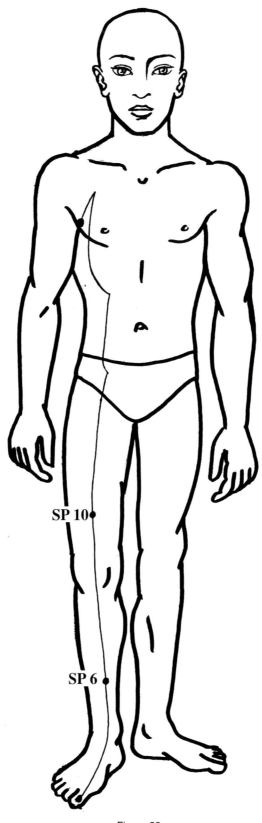

SP 10

SP 6

Figure 33

SPLEEN / PANCREAS MERIDIAN (Yin)

The spleen acts as a primary vessel of the mother earth force. Resources, stamina, immunity, and the power of grounded female nurturing energy are represented in the flow of this meridian.

Safe? Embraced?
Fill, Quench, Soothe, Nourish
Feeling Love's Lullaby
                                    SK

SP #6 - San Yin Kyo (Intersection of 3 Yin Meridians) - four fingers above the ankle on the inside of the leg on the soft ridge medial to the tibia.

Therapy for: Female reproductive problems, inducing labor (exercise great caution in pregnancy), insomnia, weight problems, nocturnal emission, impotence, abdominal bloating. It is the women's general health point.

SP #10 - Ketsu Kai (Ocean of Blood) - on the inside of the leg, 2 cun above the patella.

Therapy for: Female reproductive problems, insomnia, digestion, assimilation, knee problems, itching, hives.

HEART MERIDIAN

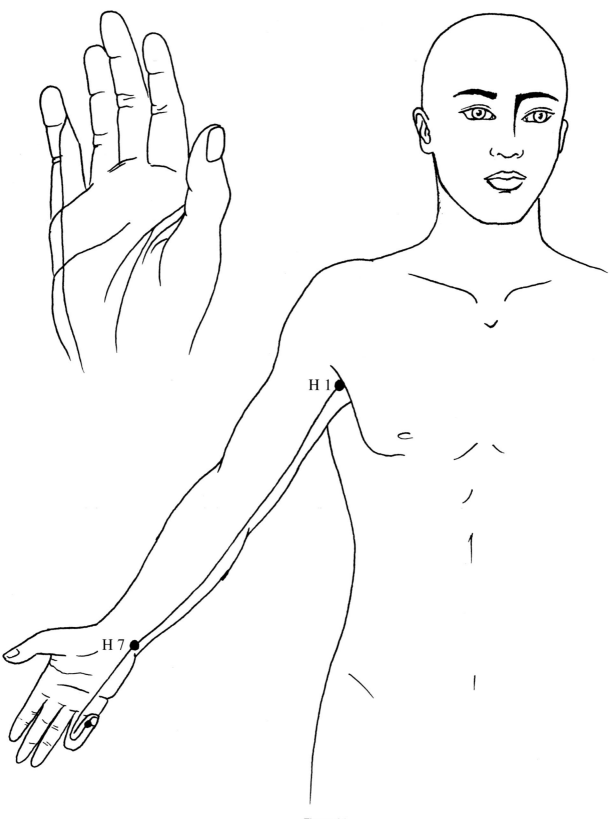

Figure 34

HEART MERIDIAN (Yin)

The heart powers the flow of blood, which feeds, energizes and inspires the life of every cell. Each cell, in turn, remembers and *"emotes"* the energy of all life experiences. The heart governs our most outward charismatic expression of the *"Human Spirit"*.

In Laughter I swell
In tears I fulfill
Express from my overflow
As a flower's petals spread
We Smile
Our Souls wink – understood
A song of joy
SK

H #1- Kyo Kusen (First Draining Point of Spring) - under the armpit (center of the achillea) medial to the auxiliary artery.

Therapy for: Arm pains, paralysis, and deficient lactation.

H #7 - Shin Mon (Gate of God) - in the crease of ulnar side of the wrist (palmar surface).

Therapy for: Palpitations, emotional release, blood pressure, and equilibrium.

Note: Some traditions assert that because the heart meridian was so vulnerable it is preferable to stimulate other meridians to effect the heart.

SMALL INTESTINE MERIDIAN

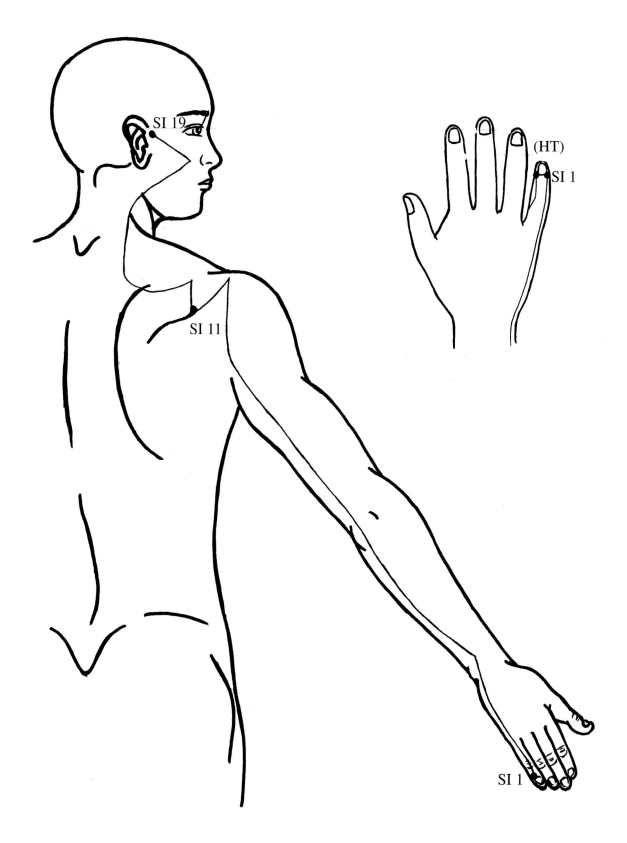

Figure 35

SMALL INTESTINE MERIDIAN (Yang)

The small intestine assimilates and converts the majority of our daily food into a form the body can use. In addition to what we eat, the body's fuel encompasses also what we assimilate in the myriad of our daily experiences. Thus, our ability to understand the relevancy of our emotions, and the divine inspiration they represent, is expressed and influenced by the small intestine.

O'how confused was I - Anxiety
Was it this or that
The source of pain?
Like the jaws of a steel trap
In a moment of exhaustion
A reason surfaces...
I understand
Wisdom held my hand
SK

SI #1 - Sho Taku (Beginning of the Stream) - outside the nail of the little finger (ulnar side).

Therapy for: Headache, eye problems, and lactation deficiency.

SI #11 - Ten So (Center of Heaven) - in the center of the scapula (between thoracic vertebrae 4 and 5.

Therapy for: Shoulder pain, overeating, and relief from accumulated mental tension.

SI #19 - Chyo Ku (Palace of Hearing) - in the depression between the mandibular joint and the tragus (just in front of the middle section of the ear.)

Therapy for: Ear ringing, sinus headache, and sexual frustration.

BLADDER MERIDIAN

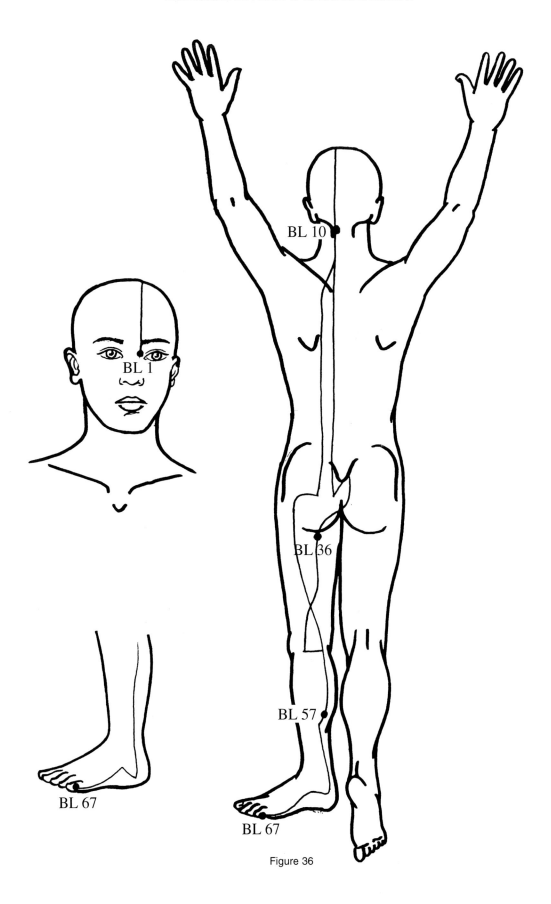

Figure 36

BLADDER MERIDIAN (Yang)

This is the longest meridian in the body. It generates the power to eliminate wastes through urination and circulates the body's *"internal essence"* energy through the whole body via the central nervous system. Bladder network circulates the energetic *elixir* of our fundamental structures (bones, marrow, and brain). Bladder meridian clarifies and further motivates our responses in *flowing* through changes.

"Boldly going where none have been before"*
Catch the moment,
The starter's signal...the Sound
Charged, Motivated, Primed.
SK

BL #1 - Sei Mei (Bright Light) - in the crease found between the eye and the bridge of the nose.

Therapy for: Tired eyes, vision problems, facial paralysis, sinuses.

BL #10 - Ten Chu (Pillar of Heaven) - alongside the first cervical vertebrae.

Therapy for: Headache, vision problems, neck stiffness, nasal obstruction.

BL #36 - Fu Bun (Divided Appendix) - midpoint where the leg and buttocks meet.

Therapy for: Paralysis, sciatica, backache

BL #57 - Shyo Zan (In the Mountains) - midway on the calf muscle (gastrocnemius).

Therapy for: Varicose veins, leg cramps, paralysis, tired legs.

BL #67 - Shi Yin (Extreme Yin) - outside edge of the nail in the little toe.

Therapy for: Difficulty in labor, malposition of fetus.

*Reference Gene Rodenberry, Star Trek author.

The points BL #13 through BL #28 are especially valuable in assessing and addressing indications related to various organ and meridian stagnation. They are called the associated *"yu"* points. They transport *"energy/chi"* to the internal organs. (See the following diagram).

YU POINTS

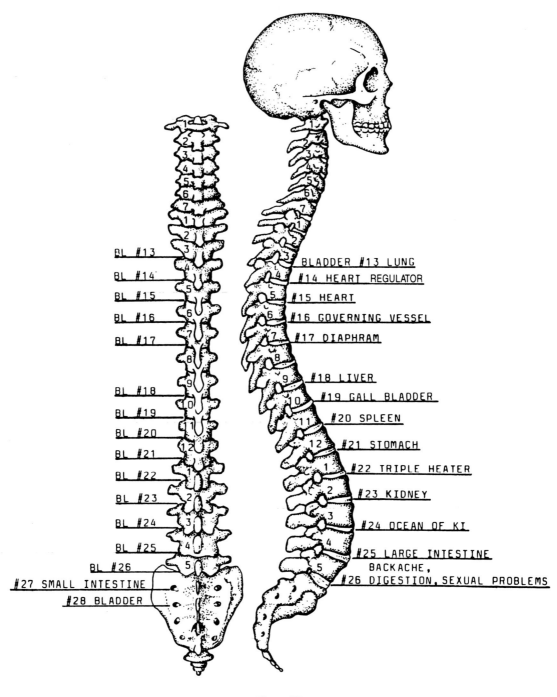

Figure 37

KIDNEY MERIDIAN

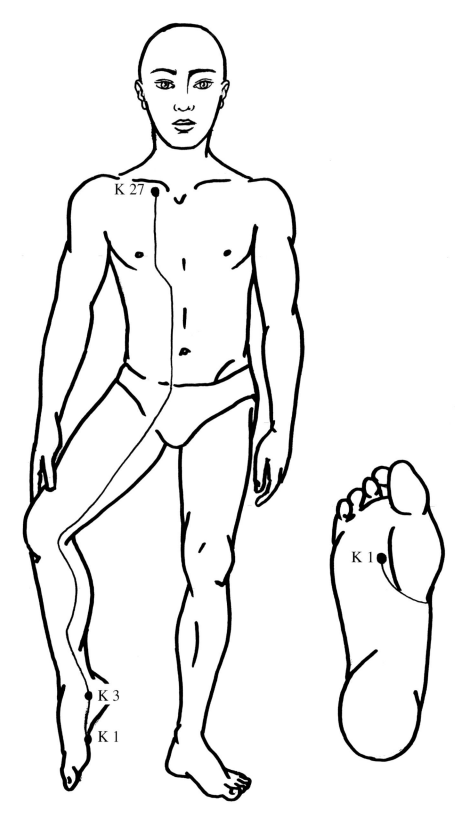

Figure 38

KIDNEY MERIDIAN (Yin)

In Chinese philosophy, the Kidneys do more than filter the blood. They also store the body's internal essence energy, called *"Jing chi"*. This elixir is the source of our pre- and post-natal energetic reserves. Our reservoir of *"Jing"* is directly linked to reproductive/sexual functions and the creative source of universal consciousness.

In the depths of the unknown
Lies a Sound, The echo of a voice
A Destiny Profound
Follow its call! I choose
Stretch, take a chance
Play it safe? I'd rather dance
SK

K #1 - Yu Sen (Bubbling Spring) - midway on the sole of the foot in the depression between, and 2 1/2 cun below, the second and third toe.

Therapy for: Epilepsy, headache, nausea, and menstrual pains.

K #3- Tai Kei (Great Groove) - in the depression halfway between the medial malleolus and the Achilles tendon.

Therapy for: All kidney disorders, nocturnal emission, menstrual problems, and paralysis in lower extremities.

K #27 - Yu Fu (Palace of Transportation) - in the depression between the clavicle and the first rib, 2 cun from the midline of the chest.

Therapy for: Asthma, cough, and vomiting.

HEART REGULATOR MERIDIAN

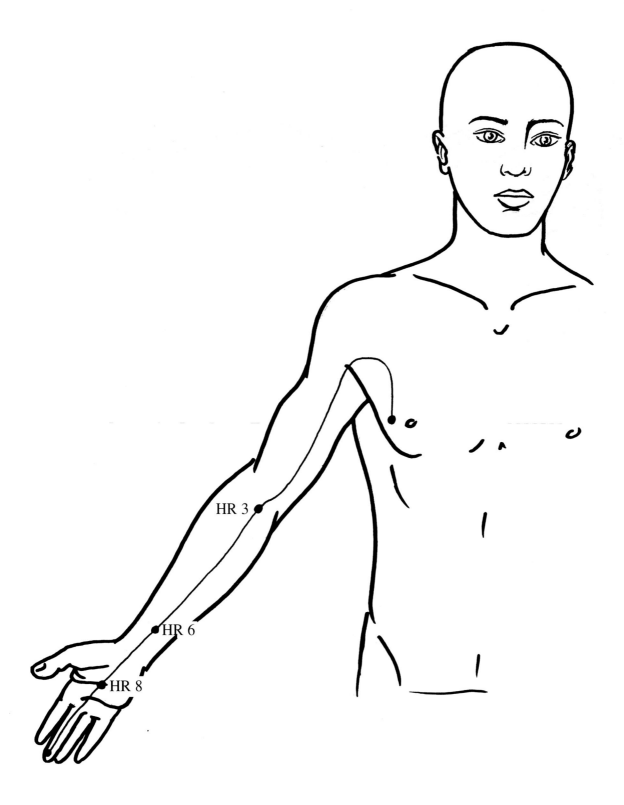

Figure 39

HEART REGULATOR

The Heart Regulator (also called Pericardium) assists and protects the heart. It acts as a buffer for pain sensitivity and as a helper in circulatory functions. In extreme cases of heart disorders (physically or emotionally) the heart regulator may offer an alternative for therapy. Sometimes called *"Supplemental Fire"*, the Heart Regulator is like a gateway, regulating the fuel to the *"absolute"* fire (heart).

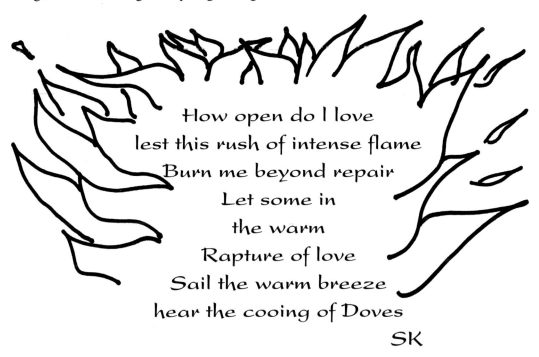

How open do I love
lest this rush of intense flame
Burn me beyond repair
Let some in
the warm
Rapture of love
Sail the warm breeze
hear the cooing of Doves

SK

HR #3 - Kyoku Taku (in the crease) - on the palmar surface of the elbow, on the ulnar side of the tendon.

Therapy for: Angina, fever, palpitations.

HR #6-Nei Kan (Inside Gate) - between the tendons 2 inches above the wrist fold.

Therapy for: Vomiting, insomnia, palpitations, chest pains.

HR #8 - Ro Kyu (Palace of Turmoil) - in the middle of the palm, between the middle and ring fingers.

Therapy for: Exhaustion, anxiety, epilepsy, and hic-cough.

TRIPLE HEATER MERIDIAN

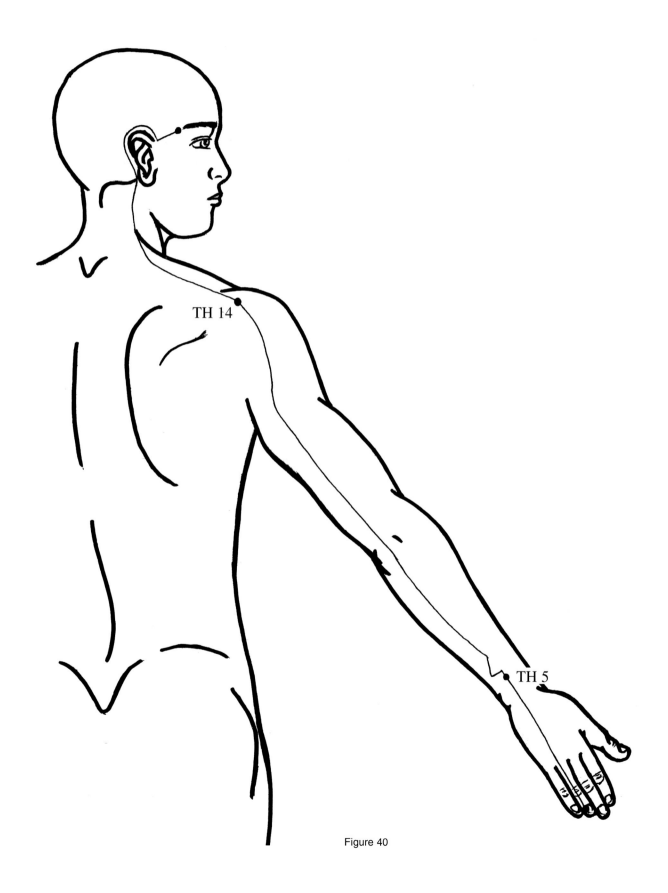

Figure 40

TRIPLE HEATER MERIDIAN (Yang)

The Triple Heater circulates heat and protection for the body. Its fuel is provided by assimilated food from the Small Intestine*, the body's storage of Kidney *"Jing Chi"*, and *"Lung/Air"* Chi. The Triple Heater circulates emotional charge and healing resulting from expressions of the heart, heart regulator and small intestine to the, 1) upper, 2) middle, or, 3) lower body. In regard to triple heater assessment, I would like to offer a simple method which can be added to meridian, back and hara palpitation. Hold one palm over the, 1) lower *Hara* or back, 2) *solar plexus* area and, 3) upper chest/clavicle area to feel which zone - lower, middle, or upper - has the least or greatest concentration of heat/energy.

*All this joy and
the harvest of my tears
searches to move
high, middle or low, let it flow
Where it lands
My Soul will know*

SK

TH #5 - Gai Kan (outer barrier) - on the dorsal surface between the radius and ulna, 2 cun above the wrist.

Therapy for: Paralysis, chest and upper back pains, colds, fever, deafness.

TH #14 - Ken Ryo (Top of the Shoulder) - upon raising the arm horizontally, TB 14 is the most posterior indentation on the shoulder (the anterior one is LI 15).

Therapy for: Paralysis, shoulder joint troubles.

*In Chinese Medicine the Spleen has similar functions to the Western Medicine's view of Small Intestine functions.

GALLBLADDER MERIDIAN

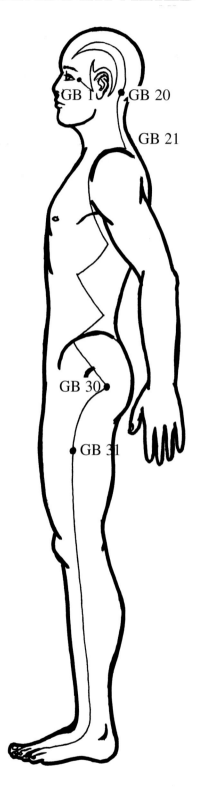

Figure 41

GALLBLADDER MERIDIAN (Yang)

The Gallbladder meridian acts as the managing official that carries out the *"foresight-ful"* plans *"masterminded"* by the Liver. It directs the Liver's *"masterplan"* through physical secretions (bile) and is associated energetically with expedient movement/action.

In form and structure the spark of True Dreams
Spontaneously directed
blood, to cells
Springs to Life
Human Consciousness takes a new step
SK

GB #1 - Do Shi Ryo (Eye Bone) - on the temple next to the eye.

Therapy for: Headache, eye troubles, and paralysis

GB #20 - Fu Chi (Pond of Wind) - in the depression under the occipital ridge, 2 cun from the center of the neck.

Therapy for: Vertigo, stiffness, colds, headache, and eye swelling.

GB #21 - Ken Sei (Well in the Shoulder) - the highest point on the shoulder, midway between the neck base and the acromion.

Therapy for: Headache, uterine bleeding, lactation difficulty, digestive disorders, neck and shoulder stiffness,.

GB #30 - Kan Chyo (Jumping Pivot) - large indentation on the hip in the gluteus maximus.

Therapy for: Sciatica, paralysis of lower extremities, lower back pain, reproductive problems.

GB #31 - Fu Shi (Market of Wind) - midpoint on the outside of the thigh.

Therapy for: Low back pain, mental anxiety, and digestive disorders.

LIVER MERIDIAN

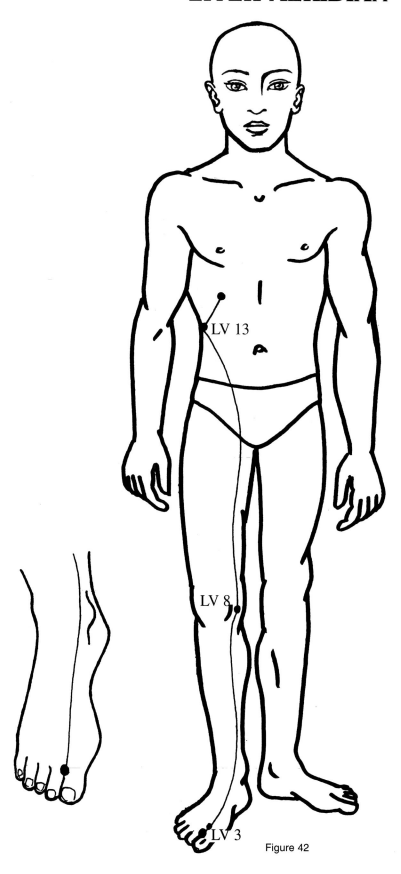

LV 13

LV 8

LV 3

Figure 42

LIVER MERIDIAN (Yin)

The multi-functional liver *"masterminds"* direction for our ideas, spontaneously plans, organizes and activates our dreams. Order, patience, or their absence, are key associations with this meridian. In comparison to the Gallbladder, the Liver directs from a more *long term or futuristic perspective.*

The Executive, The Mastermind
How quickly you Respond
Lighting your sparks,
Blowing in the winds
Fresh forever
the Spirit Transcends
SK

LV #3 - Tai Chu (Big Rush) - 2 cun up from the web between the first and second toe.

Therapy for: Headache, disorientation and balance symptoms, eye problems, and uterine bleeding.

LV #8 - Kiyoku Sen (Curved Spring) - 2 to 3 cun medial from the center of the patella (knee).

Therapy for: Urogenital troubles, impotence, hernia, and knee problems.

LV #13 - Shyo Mon (Distinguished Gate) - on the front of the body below the tip of the 11th rib.

Therapy for: Abdominal pain and vomiting.

GOVERNING VESSEL MERIDIAN

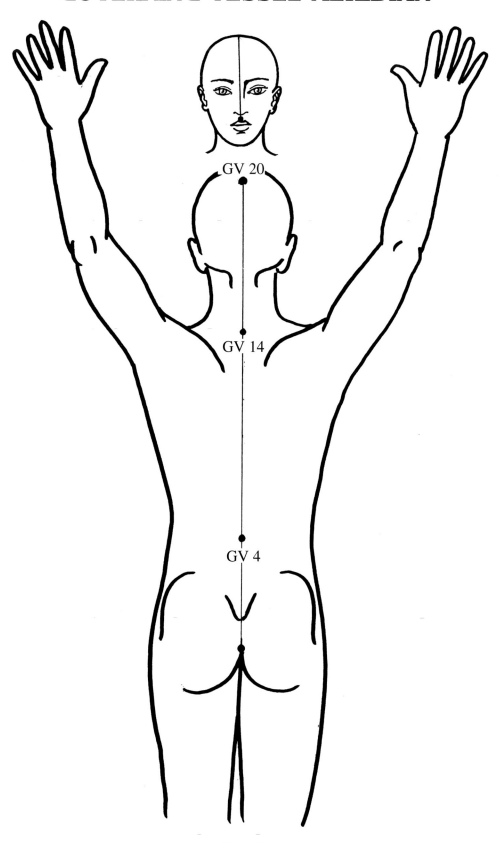

Figure 43

GOVERNING VESSEL MERIDIAN (Yang)

One of the *"extra ordinary"* unilateral channels, the Governing Vessel, is the internal manifestation and generator of heaven's force, that directly communicates the energy emanating through the seven chakras.

GV #4 - Mei Mon (Gate of Life) - between lumbar vertebrae 2 and 3 on the spinous processes.

Therapy for: Lumbago, spermatorrhea, impotence.

GV #14 - Dai Tsui (Big Vertebrae) - between the 7th cervical vertebra and the 1st thoracic vertebra.

Therapy for: Fever, colds, allergies, asthma.

GV #20 - Hya Kue (One Hundred Meetings) - on the midline, on top of the skull, in line with the upper edge of the ears.

Therapy for: Headaches, dizziness, hemorrhoids, epilepsy.

CONCEPTION VESSEL MERIDIAN

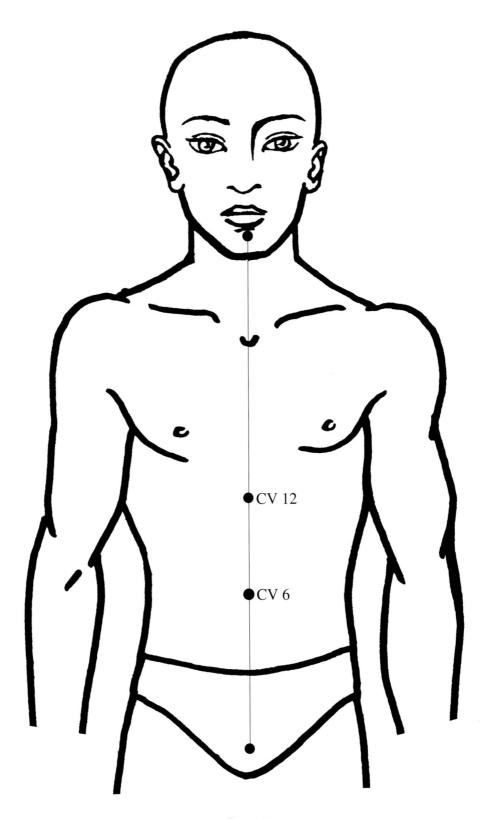

Figure 44

CONCEPTION VESSEL MERIDIAN (Yin)

Another *"extra ordinary"* channel, the Conception Vessel, receives and generates earth's force, and complements the Governing Vessel in circulating the essence that emanates from the seven chakras.

CV #6 - Ki Kai (Ocean of Energy) - 1½ inches below the navel.

Therapy for: Lack of vitality, cramps, diarrhea, uterine bleeding, nocturnal emission, menstruation difficulties.

CV #12 - Chu Kan (Midway) - in the soft part of the solar plexus approximately four inches above the navel.

Therapy for: Nausea, general abdominal and digestive stagnation.

The following diagram (figure 45) shows the *"BO"* or *"Alarm"* points. Heightened sensitivity with pain usually indicates an acute challenge in the associated organ.

BO POINTS
(Alarm)

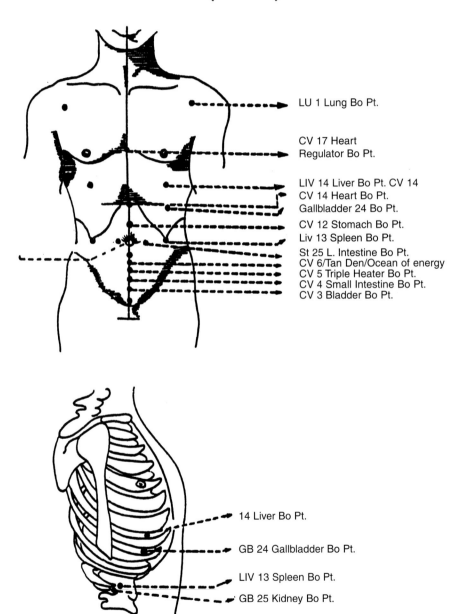

LU 1 Lung Bo Pt.

CV 17 Heart
Regulator Bo Pt.

LIV 14 Liver Bo Pt. CV 14
CV 14 Heart Bo Pt.
Gallbladder 24 Bo Pt.

CV 12 Stomach Bo Pt.
Liv 13 Spleen Bo Pt.

St 25 L. Intestine Bo Pt.
CV 6/Tan Den/Ocean of energy
CV 5 Triple Heater Bo Pt.
CV 4 Small Intestine Bo Pt.
CV 3 Bladder Bo Pt.

14 Liver Bo Pt.

GB 24 Gallbladder Bo Pt.

LIV 13 Spleen Bo Pt.

GB 25 Kidney Bo Pt.

Figure 45

The preceding indications for therapy are examples from which we can begin observation and verification derived from our own personal experiences. Energy can stagnate at any number of points along any meridian. Furthermore, energetic activation and healing influences can be triggered from any number of points.

Therapy dynamics manifest differently with each person we work with. Oftentimes, results are more dependent on *how* we work, rather than the points we stimulate. The unique energy quality of the practitioner communicating and connecting with each client is of the ultimate importance. Profound transformations result when the practitioner *empathizes* or develops a *communion* with the essence of each client portrayed in the *feeling* present at every point, meridian or area. Eventually intuition becomes our best guide. The points will show themselves, and a wealth of teachings, experiences and great satisfaction will adorn the work.

In addition to the most popularly utilized six meridian pairs, there are also eight "extra" channels which run throughout the body, connecting at various points along the already mentioned meridian lines. (The governing and conception vessels are two of the eight extra channels.) Various forms of Asian bodywork and acupuncture integrate the *extraordinary* channels, *internal meridian* pathways, *tendinomuscle* channels, *cutaneous* regions, and *connecting* meridians into their work. Also, the late Shizuto Masunaga described in great detail variations on the locations of the traditional meridian lines. The applications of these systems have great value and if you are interested, I recommend the *Essentials of Chinese Acupuncture* and *Zen Shiatsu* for further study.

MERIDIAN THERAPY

Some theories suggest that stimulating a meridian along its natural direction of flow (i.e. on a *yin* meridian, move up from foot to head, or on a *yang* meridian, move down from head to foot) creates a tonifying effect, while going against the meridian's natural direction creates a sedating/dispersing effect. Also, slower techniques with more holding create tonification through nurturing, while quicker, sharper techniques initiate sedation and dispersion. Let experience be your teacher. Find what works for you. I maintain that working the meridians intuitively with a minimum of analysis reveals the best location, direction, duration, and quality of touch to be used. Trust your feelings, and discover what results are obtained.

As mentioned previously, working the meridians at distal points from the actual difficulty can be very effective. A typical example is in severe neck pain, caused by "whiplash". Direct stimulation on the neck could aggravate this extreme situation. Working the legs or feet, however, will generate a flow of energy, either toward or away from the neck, thus promoting a condition where neck relief is obtained through indirect stimulation.

It is also important to comprehend that any difficulty, indication, or disease could be caused and most effectively transformed by stimulation of *any* meridian. For example, "bladder pain" could be traced back to inefficient liver or large intestine energy or an emotional problem affecting the heart and blood circulation. Finding the source is the key to changing the condition. In the meantime, as experience with assessment and therapy is developing just observe the meridians and points with their Empty and Full qualities. Connect with the client at these places, allowing the body to become a facilitator of beneficial movement and change.

What to Do?

How Can I Help?

Let Go of a Result

Be there, Breathe

Honor the Space - Healing Proceeds

SK

HANDS-ON TECHNIQUES

The Elbow

The elbow can be a very powerful tool for initiating change. For people who respond to deep penetration, elbow pressure is ideal, especially in some of those tough, harder areas. The following photos show some practical elbow applications.

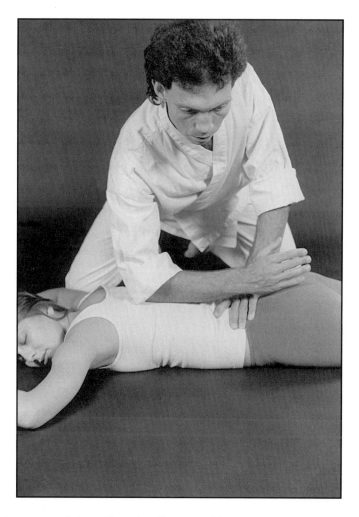

In an extended position, the elbow provides a more subtle effect.

To obtain a sharper, more penetrating effect, simply bend the arm toward you. This allows the edge of the ulna to focus on the point or the area you are working. Because of its potential strength, bend your arm slowly while listening carefully for how well the additional pressure is being received. Also, exert more pressure with your mother hand, before you increase the elbow pressure.

Your center of gravity sinks by spreading your knees. This will increase the pressure by lowering the body instead of using the arm muscles.

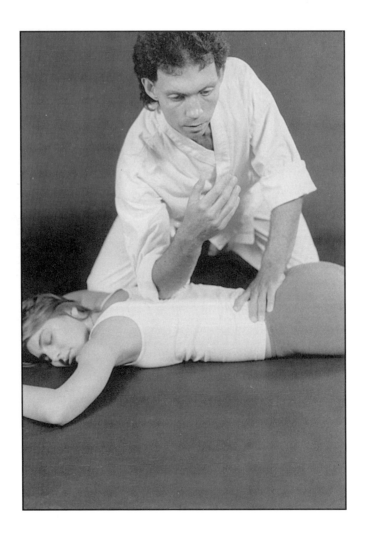

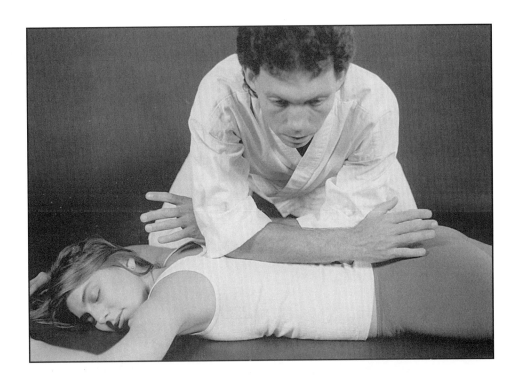

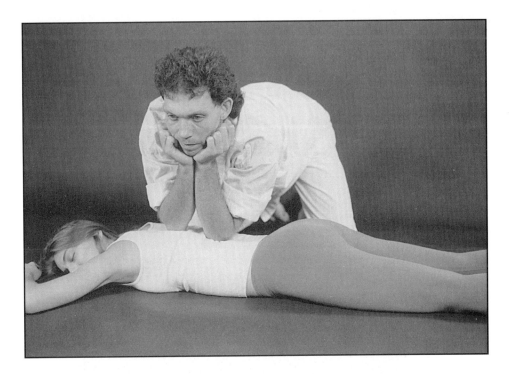

A very effective technique is accomplished by **slowly** penetrating the tissue layers with both elbows side by side. When applied sensitively, with equal pressure from both elbows, the practitioner is well received without causing any pain.

Additional elbow techniques:

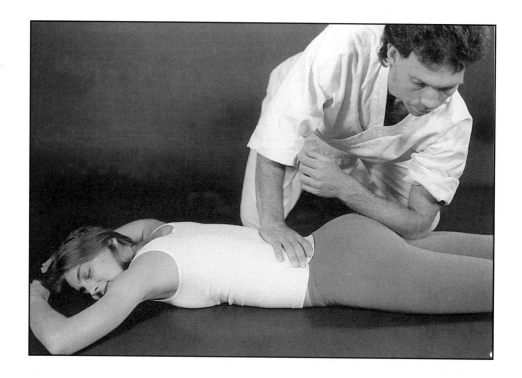

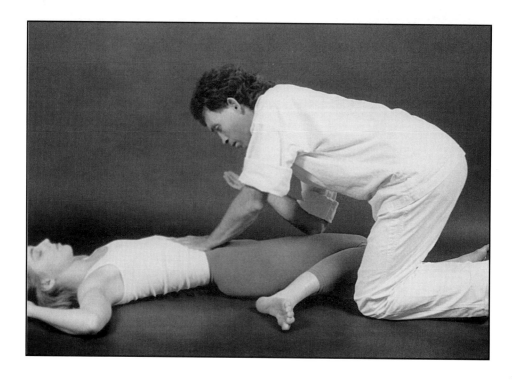

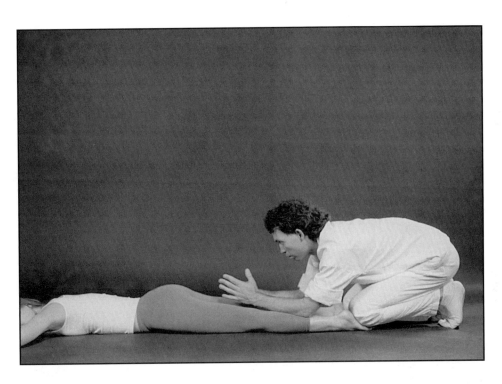

The elbows create a closer physical and energetic connection with the potential to initiate extreme physical or emotional changes/reactions. Sensitivity, clarity and compassion are essential.

THE KNEE

The knees are very helpful in moving energy throughout the larger areas of the body, like the thighs and buttocks. They are particularly handy when the client responds agreeably to substantial contact. When well utilized, our entire weight can be focused on an area through the knees creating a feeling of great support without any pain.

Put one hand on the lower back, and the other hand on the lower leg. Use your hands to support and regulate your weight as you gradually place your knee into your client's thighs. By using your hands to support your weight, excess pressure from the knees is avoided. This technique can be done prone or supine.

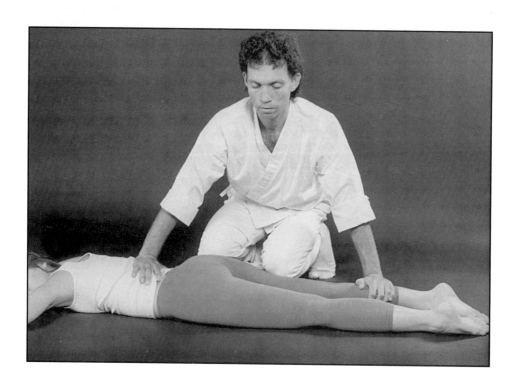

Stomach Meridian with Knees

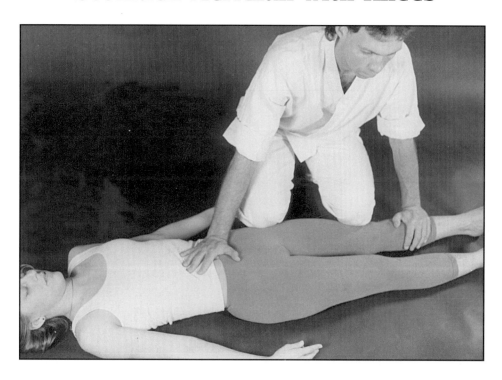

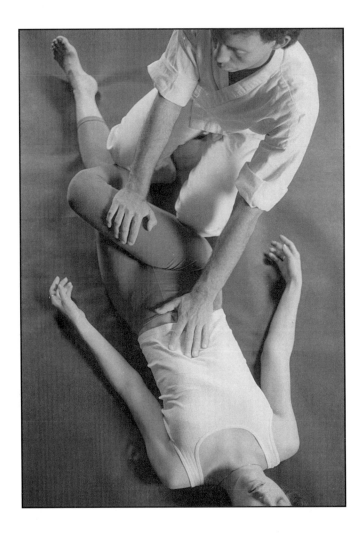

The following are some other possible knee techniques. They require more sensitivity to determine which clients will "receive" them.

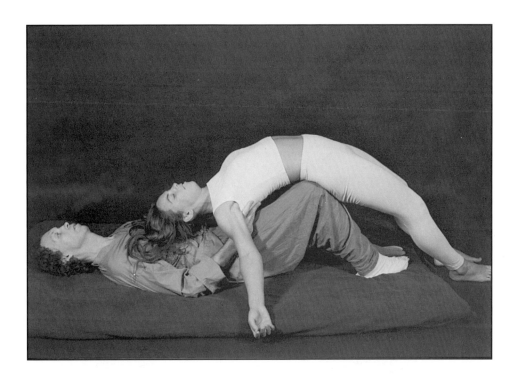

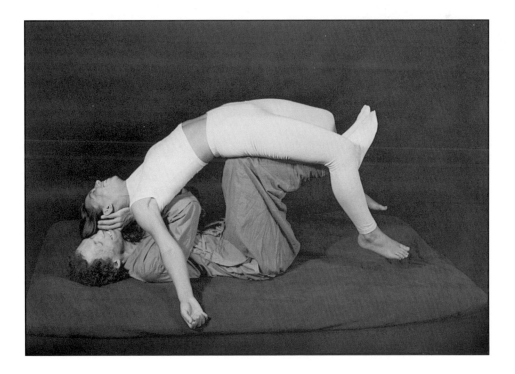

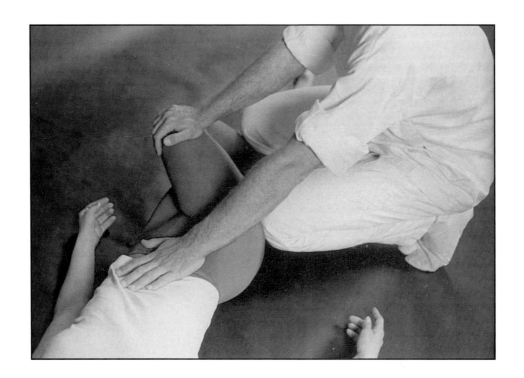

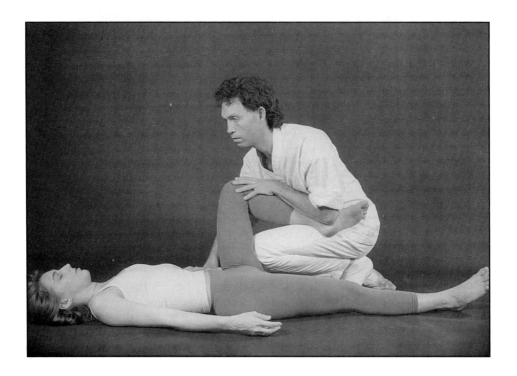

THE FEET

Shown below are some simple techniques using the feet. I recommend Shizuko Yamamoto's book *Barefoot Shiatsu and Family Health Care* for more information on this style.

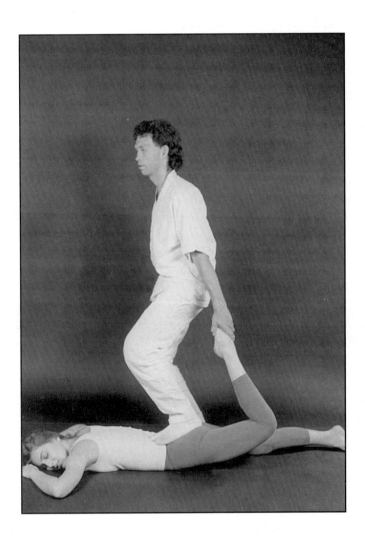

As client exhales, lean forward while pulling their leg toward you. This opens the hip socket, stretches the lower back and stomach meridian (on the front of the legs). Be mindful of directing the sacrum towards the feet which lengthens the spine instead of contracting it.

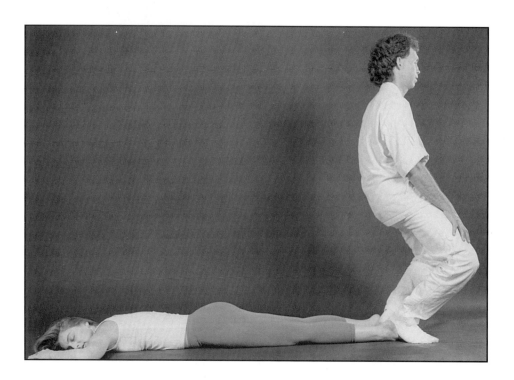

As your body weight drops, deeper stimulation is initiated on the client's feet.

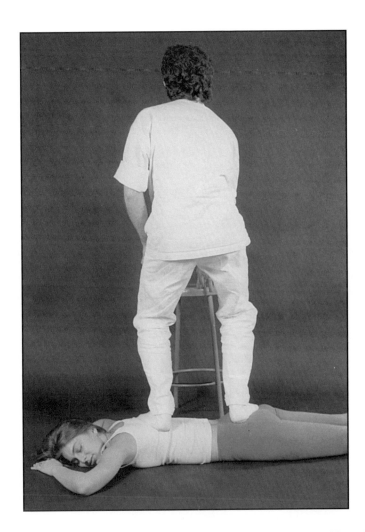

As client exhales, shift weight into the upper back. On the inhale, shift to the sacrum. Do this quickly to stimulate respiration and blood/energy flow. Support from the chair will regulate a comfortable amount of weight for the client.

THE SHOULDER and UPPER BACK AREA

The shoulder and upper back areas act as a protector for the underlying organs, the heart and the lungs. Because of the sturdier nature of the bones and muscles in this area, it is natural for the body to shift its pains and tensions here rather than house them in the more vulnerable areas, like the lower back and abdomen. To alleviate pain in the shoulders, it is equally, if not more important, to also tonify or strengthen the vulnerable places in order to effect long-lasting results. Zen-Touch™ therapy suggests that this Empty area was the original source of the pain, which traveled to the more obvious Full area. Thus, therapy is most effectively focused on the "Low/Empty" rather than on the symptomatic "High/Full."

Connecting the high with the low initiates a long-awaited body balancing effect.

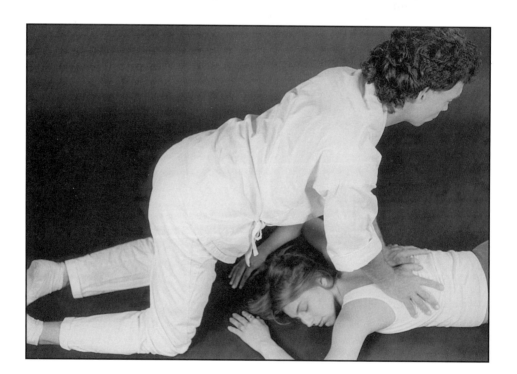

THE NECK

Sensitivity in the neck is common because it is a gathering place for most of the meridians and it has a high concentration of blood circulation and nerve endings. The neck also represents the bridge or connection between mind and body. Compromised communication between thinking and acting are a common cause for tension commonly held here.

Applying therapy on the neck requires great sensitivity. In every technique we use, it is essential for our clients to feel totally supported. This support initiates a trust, which creates deep relaxation, and long-lasting effects. Compassion and sensitivity toward each client is essential. Some people's necks require a slow, light approach, while others require deep and penetrating techniques. Be open to a wide possibility of variations.

The best results occur when the client feels so well supported that they surrender control of all the muscles in their neck. At this point, it actually feels as though the neck and head are like a loosely rotating ball that the client is enjoyably letting the practitioner play with. This feeling can be achieved more often when mobilization of the neck originates from *Hara* motion, rather than hand movement only. Clients will be more likely to trust and surrender control when they feel this deep body support.

The therapy tempo is also crucially important. A slow approach usually works well when working with people whose necks are stiff and tight, while a faster tempo *may* be effective for clients who allow their necks to relax completely.

An effective technique for clients who keep control of their neck movement is to move very, very **slowly** without using any consistency or obvious pattern in the direction of motion. The client will stop anticipating the practitioner's next move and allow her neck to flow.

The following demonstrate some very effective neck techniques:

Cervical Rock

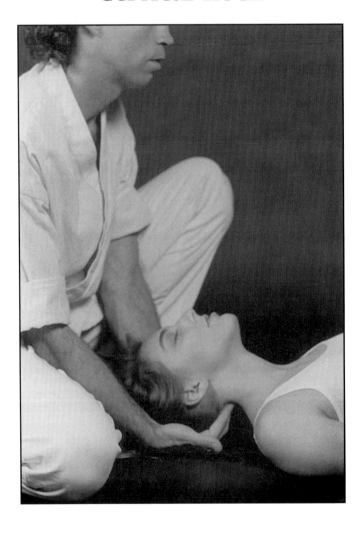

Side Stretch

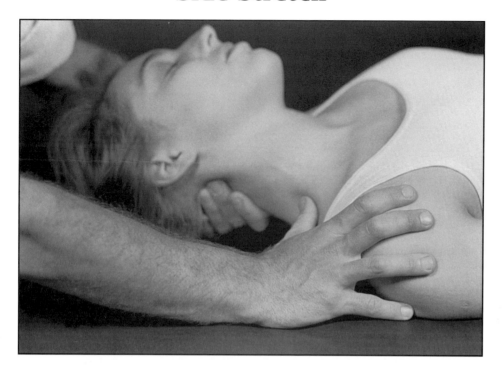

Sternocleidomastoid Stimulation

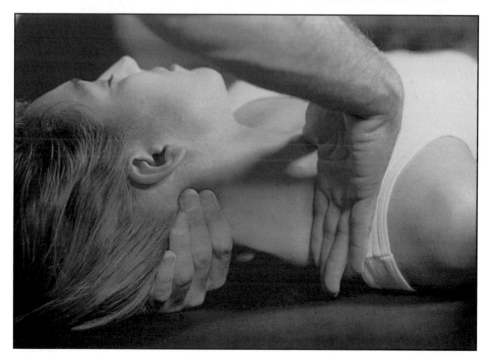

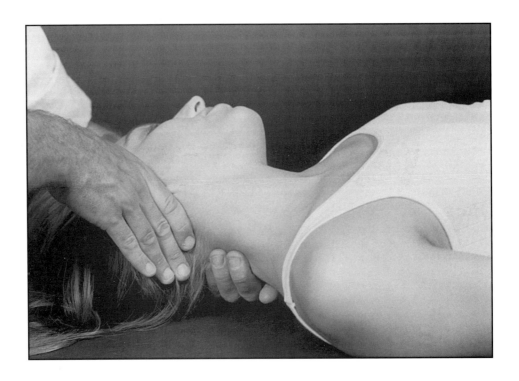

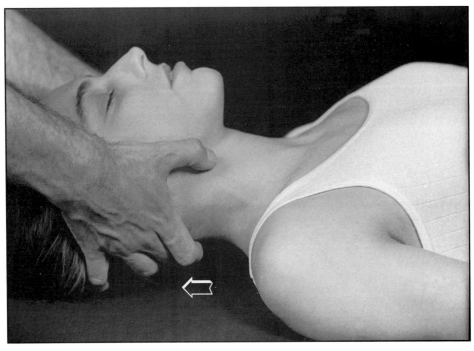

Cervical Pull (Traction)

ASSESSMENT

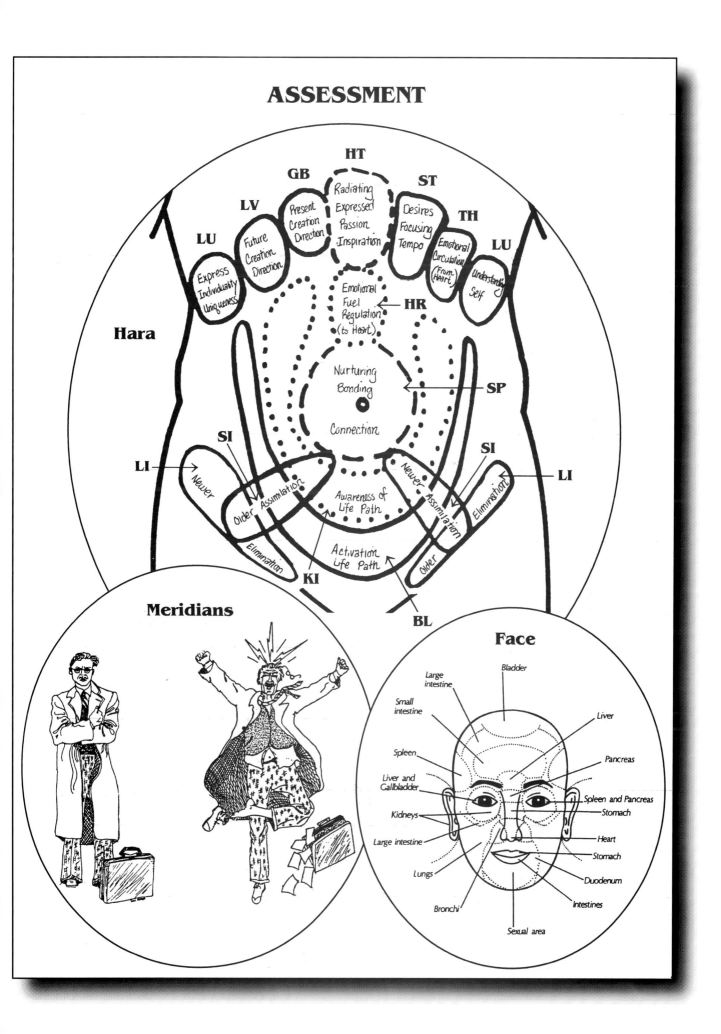

ASSESSMENT

As we are learning to intuitively feel which areas need attention, it is helpful, and for most of us essential, to develop by starting with some practical tools. In addition to the *meridians, tsubos,* the *chakras*, and the five *transformations* systems, I will offer some new possibilities:

BACK ASSESSMENT

Because the back of the body is harder and more steadfast than the front, older and more chronic tendencies are often revealed here. For example, patterns of stagnation that have been going on since youth might show themselves in the condition of the back. Sensitivities in the associated points, listed in Figure 37 (pg. 86) guide us to which meridians or organs require attention. Also, the diagram in Figure 46 (pg. 125) can be useful as a further assessment tool.

Discolorations, pains, hot and cold areas, protrusions, indentations, Empty and Full places found in the corresponding assessment areas can all direct our sessions. These signs relate to the meridians, organs, and their associated physical, psychological and spiritual qualities.

Another important Traditional concept integrated into Zen Touch™ is that assessment and therapy are inseparable. As we touch stagnated areas, they begin to change. The rate at which they resist or change is an indication of their seriousness. Thus, therapy and assessment show themselves simultaneously.

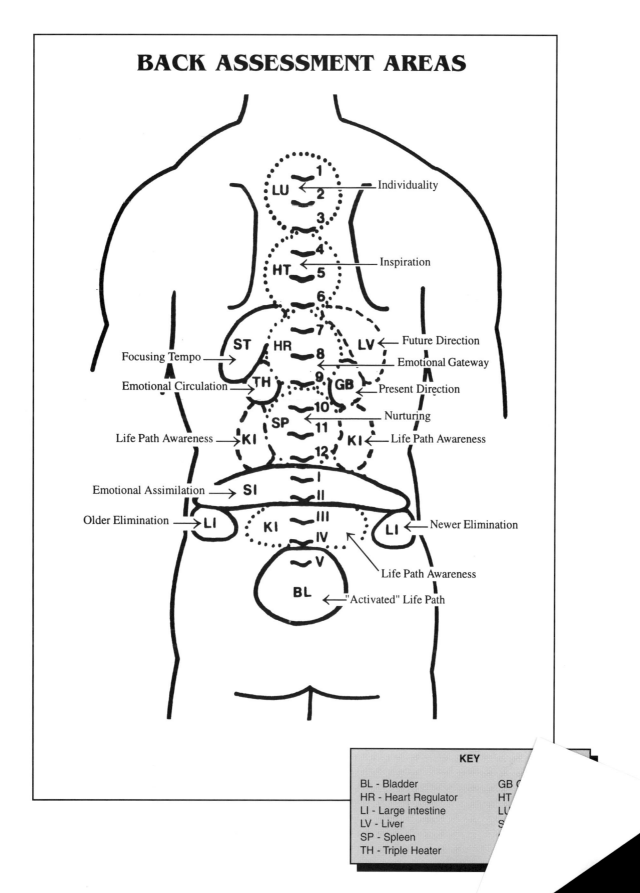

BACK ASSESSMENT AREAS

Individuality

Inspiration

Future Direction

Focusing Tempo — Emotional Gateway

Emotional Circulation — Present Direction

Nurturing

Life Path Awareness — Life Path Awareness

Emotional Assimilation

Older Elimination — Newer Elimination

Life Path Awareness

"Activated" Life Path

KEY

BL - Bladder   GB
HR - Heart Regulator   HT
LI - Large intestine   LU
LV - Liver   S
SP - Spleen
TH - Triple Heater

Figure 46

FACIAL ASSESSMENT

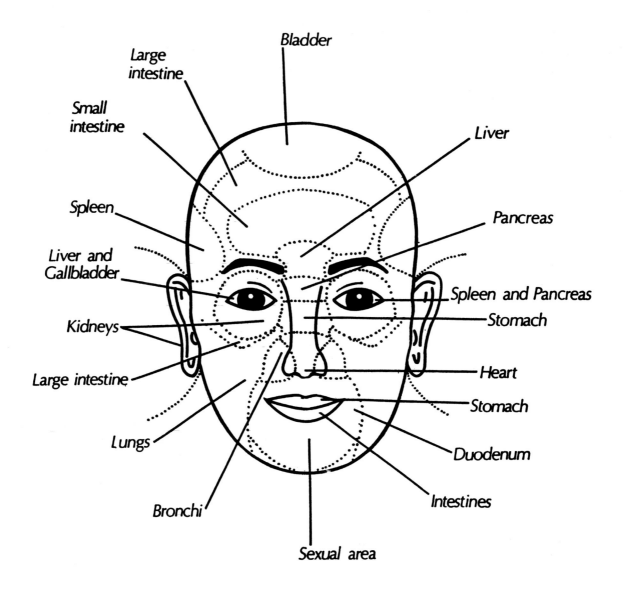

Figure 47

FACIAL ASSESSMENT

The art of physiognomy originated in China thousands of years ago. Figure 47 (pg. 126) demonstrates the areas on the face that correspond to the different organs and meridians. The subtle possibilities that exist extend far beyond the scope of this book. The location of discoloration, irregular protrusions or indentations, swellings, dryness and any intuitive visual impressions can all be indicators of areas that require attention. Remember to consider the behavioral characteristics associated to any area that is drawing your attention.

MERIDIAN ASSESSMENT

I find that the meridians reveal energetic information, which pertains to the most recent influences affecting the client. For example, Back and Hara lung assessment areas might reveal *Emptiness* in the lungs, while the meridian itself might be tight and *Full*. The situation might be revealing how a chronic weakness is causing the meridian to over work in an effort to circulate energy to the lungs. Therapy could include *dispersion* of the *Full* lung meridian in the arm, and *tonification* of the *Empty* assessment areas. While pains, numbness, discoloration, stiffness and limited motion are all possible indications to note, remember our fundamental guideline for assessment is: *Empty* areas like to receive stimulation and *Full* areas resist and often push the practitioner away.

HARA ASSESSMENT

The *Hara* is the soft abdominal area below the rib cage and above the pubic bone. All our life essential digestive and reproductive organs are found here. The *Hara* houses the effects of all our life experiences. It reflects more of our recent life condition, in comparison to the back, which reveals more of our past influences. For example, *current* digestive troubles and/or emotional stress may be more easily observed in the *Hara* than in the back.

There are many different systems and variations of the assessment areas found in the *Hara*. In addition to the anatomical location of the internal organs Figure 26 (pg.62), we also have Figure 48 (pg. 130), which represents a system of *Hara* assessment, first observed by Shizuto Masunaga. Both physical and psychological patterns may reveal themselves at the corresponding areas, shown in either of these figures. Physical blockages may require deeper penetration, while psychological patterns may be revealed and worked with a more superficial touch.

When stimulating or assessing the *Hara*, one hand (palm) will stay stationary, acting as a supporting mother hand, while *gently* using the fingers of our other hand to sense the condition of the different assessment areas.

Because of the *Hara's* soft and vulnerable nature, it is of the utmost importance for the practitioner to initiate and maintain a feeling of trust. This is achieved by moving slowly and compassionately throughout the various assessment areas. An obtrusive or probing technique creates resistance, which masks the client's energetic condition. If the client feels tense or uncomfortable, the practitioner may, at most, manage to feel some physical dynamics. With a lack of client receptivity the likelihood of perceiving underlying "extra sensory phenomena" is greatly reduced.

The *Hara* is my personal guide to the most prevalent condition of clients — whatever their behavior, body language, face, back or meridians reveal, I am always amazed at the accuracy revealed by the *Hara*. *Hara* connection lies at the core essence of Zen-Touch™ Assessment and Therapy.

Note: When palpating, use approximately the weight of a nickel coin (just enough to feel a vibration under your fingertips).

For LU, HT, HR, SP, KI, and BL areas, palpate perpendicular (90°) to the midline of the body.

For LV, GB, ST, TH, palpate perpendicular (90°) to the ribcage.

For LI, use the ulnar edge of the palm to match the shape of this area on both sides of the hara.

For SI, straighten the palm and fingers of both hands. Place the middle and ring fingers of each hand on both areas at an angle pointing toward the navel.

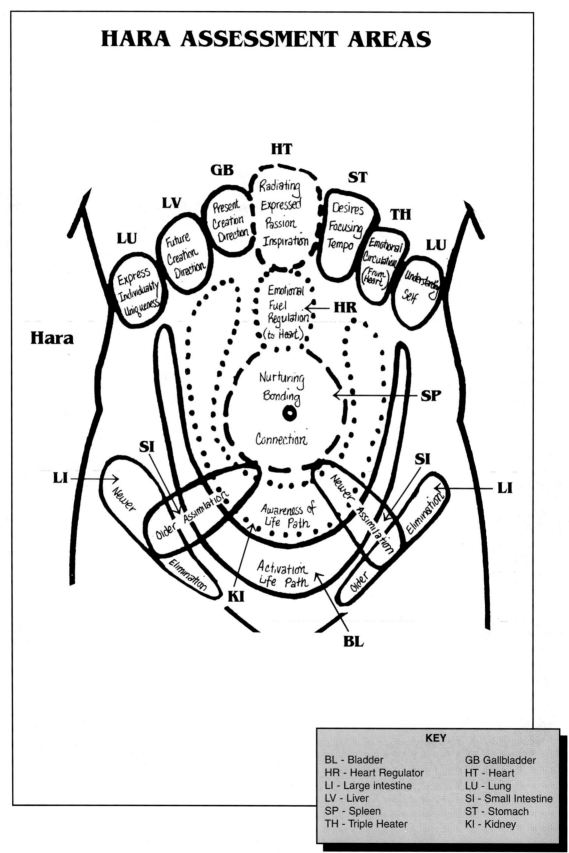

Figure 48

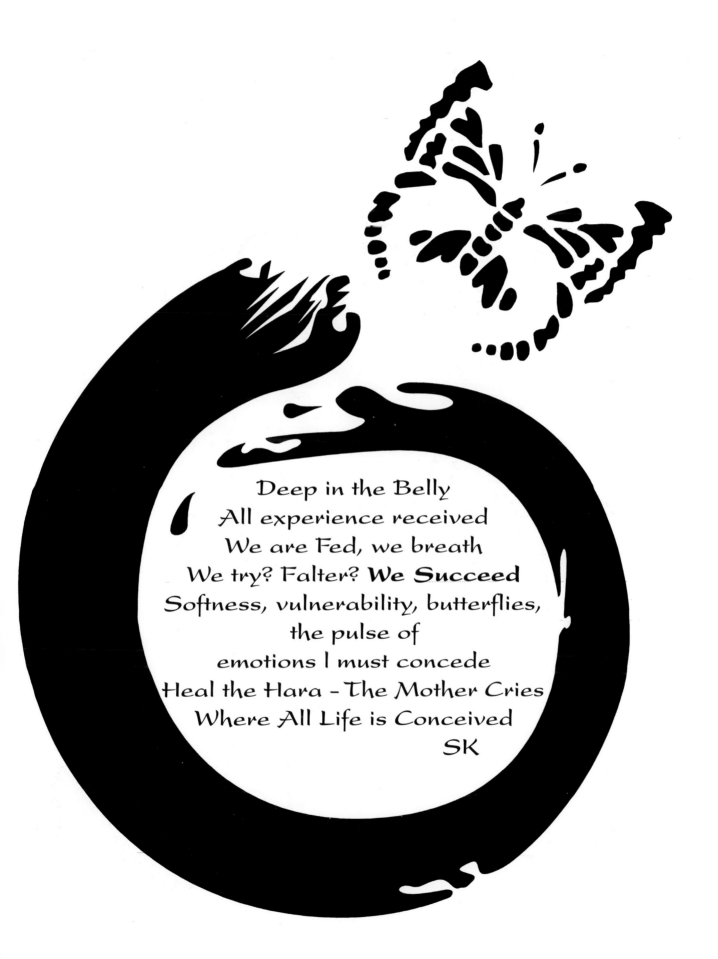

Deep in the Belly
All experience received
We are Fed, we breath
We try? Falter? **We Succeed**
Softness, vulnerability, butterflies,
the pulse of
emotions I must concede
Heal the Hara – The Mother Cries
Where All Life is Conceived
SK

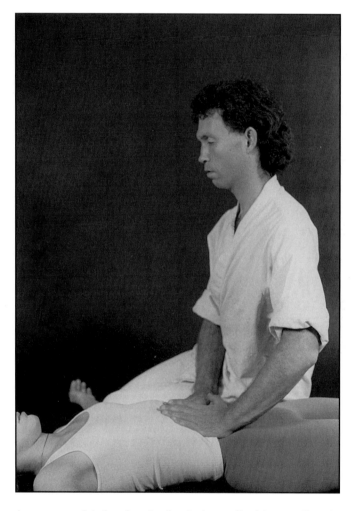

For maximum sensitivity, let the body be pulled in to client's *Hara.* This will ensure relaxation and trust...the key to revealing the client's true condition.

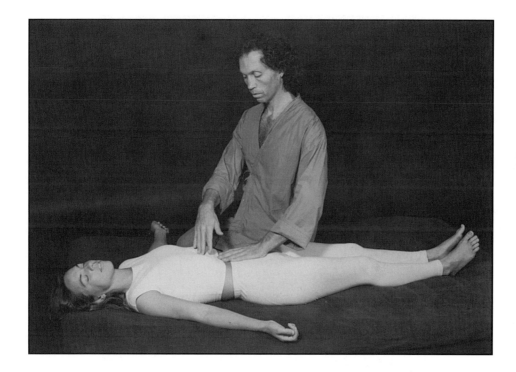

The methods mentioned represent only a few of the several assessment tools that people are using effectively all over the world. The hands, feet, tongue, ears, pulses on the wrist, sclerology, and iridology are some of the most popular. Some believe that the cells of the body are like a hologram, which stores the information of the whole throughout the different patterns of its smaller counterparts. Thus the many assessment methods are microcosms of the macrocosmic body.

Putting together all the assessment information can be a very exciting endeavor. One way to begin is by asking how your client reveals himself in relevance to the different assessment models. For example:

Yin/Yang - Is the client more passive or aggressive? Is she intellectually and philosophically oriented, or does she have more of a gutsy "go-for-it" attitude? Does he convey over-zealousness or caution? Are they a night or a day person? (Figure 10, pg. 37). Remember that the obvious front also has an equal and opposite underlying back.

The Chakras - Do you sense any behavior pattern that indicates an over-activity of one or more of the 7 Chakras? For example, are they overly talkative? When they walk, do they move from their Hara or from their shoulders? Where is her attention—higher or lower Chakras?

The Five Transformations - Does observing, listening, or touching reveal any domineering energies? You may sense that his mannerisms portray a floating or perhaps a rising energy nature. Maybe you feel that two energies, like fire and metal, play a key role in this person's lifestyle. Maybe her body mannerism evokes a nurturing or needy earth-like nature.

The Back - The look and feel of the back may offer some explanation of the past source of patterns and feelings. When you touch the back, does it feel open or resistant, protective or vulnerable? Close your eyes, empty your mind, and key words or images may materialize. Let the assessment reveal itself.

The Face - Observe the facial areas while working the Hara. Are there any correspondences or complementary associations on the face that match with what you're feeling in the Hara?

The Meridians - Perhaps the Empty-Full areas along the meridian will give you an idea of which areas are overactive or undernourished.

The Hara - Does the Hara confirm or reveal anything important? Are any emotional or physical tendencies showing themselves?

For a more detailed description, I recommend *The Book of Oriental Diagnosis, Your Face Never Lies,* by Michio Kushi, *Chinese Face Reading,* by T. Mar, *Reading the Body,* by Ohashi and my latest book, *Shaping Our Destiny: Body Reading and Recommendations for Health, Love, and Life Path.*

If we stay clear and centered, avoiding an overly analytical or dissecting approach, many profound observations will "be shown" to us. If nothing profound materializes, we can always relate to the areas as being Empty or Full; work the meridians and watch what happens.

Could it be this...
or that
to Where, to Whom, to Which
- My mind likes to chat
Let Go...Hold Breathe
Take a moment, empty
Embody Sincerity, I care
Space......
The Answer surfaces waiting where?
Right There!
Feel the current, summer heat, the cool snow
An empty vacuum draws and fills
The answer overflows
SK

Perceiving physical or psychological assessment indications is an abstract art. At a certain point of receptivity/clarity and openness, an image or perception materializes in the consciousness of the practitioner. For example, while working and sensing the nature of the Large Intestine assessment area, an image of tension or resentment over a past relationship might be *"intuited"* by the practitioner. These held feelings are both being released and observed in the Large Intestine assessment area.

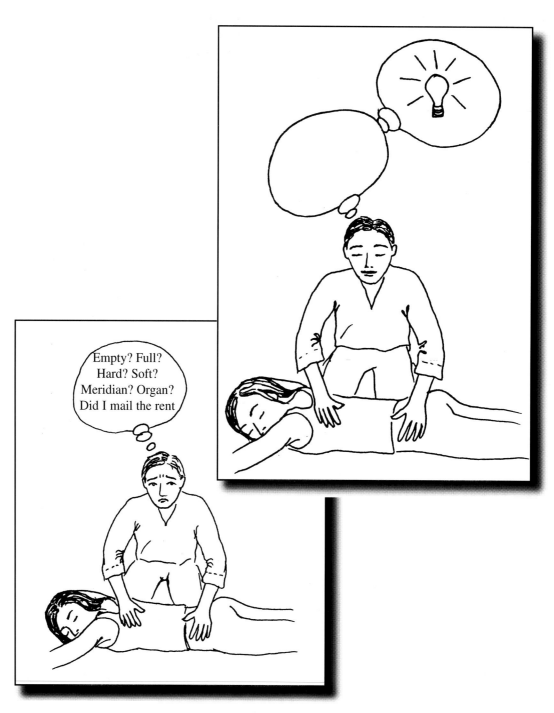

Figure 49

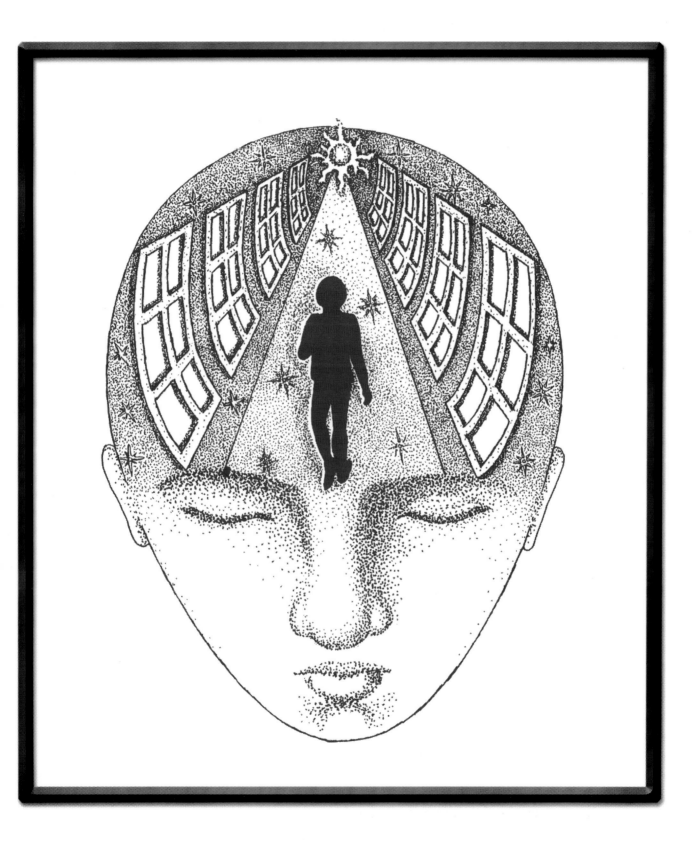

GIVING ADVICE

Recommending exercise, diet, or life style activities to clients can be of great service if they are suggested with sensitivity. The client will appreciate our concern, as long as there is no judgement or obligation attached to our advice. Also, people have different tempos at which they are willing to make changes. Some will respond to an "all or nothing" approach, while others will be more receptive if we initiate change, one step at a time. I like to check clients' *appetite* or *desire* to change. I.e., give them small *portions* of advice and watch them *hungrily* request more. In this way they choose their tempo of transformation.

Our assessment will guide us in suggesting specific individualized recommendations. For example, if you sense a constricted/metal energy influence in your client, then perhaps a "fiery exercise" like dancing or aerobics, will be effective. If their upper Chakras are overactive, contributing to a "spacey" attitude, perhaps root vegetables and grains will help to ground them.

In order to communicate better with clients, I find it very helpful for practitioners to associate key words, which describe the qualities of the conditions we perceive. For example, rather than telling clients that their lower back feels jitsu or *full*, it is more effective to describe that fullness to them, e.g., "There seems to be some tightness in your lower back." Provide words that reflect the quality of the condition and then suggest what would complement or improve the condition. "My suggestions are intended to provide warmth and a calming effect."

Also, the areas themselves can be referred to by key phrases of association, i.e., instead of referring to the kidney we use a key word or phrase like the *life awareness, willpower drive,* or *life force center.* Combining *empty* or *full* qualities with organ associations will create a deeper connection with clients, e.g., instead of saying the kidney is *jitsu*, we could ask, "Is your *willpower* and *drive in life* feeling somewhat *restless*?" On a physical level we might sense and offer to our client that their metabolic adapting functions are on overdrive and ask them if a more settled feeling would be welcome. A closer rapport with clients will result with this approach.

Encourage Clients! Using words like "bad," "stagnated," "stuck," connote negativity and often instills guilt. Instead, reinforce the *movement to wellness,* e.g., "I am suggesting that exercise, and eating more salads will promote a feeling of *freshness* in your life. Would you welcome such a feeling?"

The following chart on Zen-Touch™ Body Assessment gives some examples of possible options for replacing *kyo/empty* and *jitsu/full* in our vocabulary. I encourage everyone to describe in his or her own words/phrases the *feeling* presented by their client's condition.

ZEN-TOUCH™ BODY ASSESSMENT

	Physical/Material	Vibrational
Emptiness (Kyo) - Primal Source of Imbalance	Insufficient quantity, quality, or activity of metabolic resources or functions. Examples: Tissues, fluids, blood, lymph, hormones, nutrients, enzymes, or their movement (External/Internal imbalance is the cause). Low blood sugar causing fatigue.	• Absence • Lack • Depleted - Deficient • Exhausted • Hungry • Vacant • Seeking: • Expression • Attention • Experience • Fulfillment, manifested frequencies or life force Example: Lack of new creative expression (depleted Gallbladder [rising energy] one possible cause of frustration)

	Physical/Material	Vibrational
Over activity (Jitsu) - Indirect reaction to the unaddressed primal source of imbalance - (the Empty - Kyo)	Over abundance, over production or over activity of metabolic function, - a more obvious sign which signals the body to make adaption/rebalance. Examples: Tissues, fluids, blood, lymph, hormones, nutrients, enzymes,or their movement (External/Internal imbalance is the cause). Pain signals the body to rest or alter activity-headache (excess effect) caused by constipation (inactivity/deficient colon).	• Excess • Agitated • Excited • Restless • Hyper frequencies of Life Force Example: Anger manifests (liver-agitation) from unfulfilled desires or needs (unfulfilled/kyo stomach).

The following Zen-Touch™ Meridian Associations, Functions, and Attitudes give possible physical, emotional and mental/spiritual consciousness responses of the meridians.

ZEN-TOUCH™ MERIDIAN ASSOCIATIONS. FUNCTIONS, RESPONSES, ATTITUDES

FUNCTION	Physical	Emotional	Mental/Philosophical
KIDNEY: Life awareness, Life Force, Flow Center - "Battery"	Physical adaptability through metabolic changes.	Governs our emotional reaction to unknown (change).	Universal ideals, the big picture.
BLADDER: Life "Motivation Switch"	Purification/filtering in action.	Clarifies and further motivates our response to change.	Anticipation, incentive.
ATTITUDE: READY TO MOVE "Stoked" "Charged" (Adverse Reaction: Fear, caution, shyness, backing away, i.e., flowing back).			

FUNCTION	Physical	Emotional	Mental/Philosophical
LIVER: Command Center Mastermind	Controls and directs biotransformation of substances (pure or toxic) for energy, storage, and production.	Our directing/ commanding response to present stimuli as we see it affecting our *future*. Likes to feel "Fresh."	The power of creativity, with *future* goal in sight. Life force in form. Activated/Directed "Sparks" of the Spirit.
GALLBLADDER: Dispatchment, Chief Distributor "Switchboard Operator"	Distributor of energy.	*Present* effect of directing/commanding Likes to feel "on the up and up."	*Present* power of creative life force in form. Likes to "Discover."
ATTITUDE: ORGANIZING and DIRECTING THE LIFE FORCE, "On the Case." (Adverse Reaction: Frustration, anger).			

FUNCTION	Physical	Emotional	Mental/Philosophical
HEART: Spirit Circulation	Circulator of blood and life force.	Passionate, Inspiring	Emanation and communication of spirit and soul - the bright fires within and out.
SMALL INTESTINE: Spirit Replenisher, Assimilator	Assimilation, integration, incorporation of nutrition.	Grounding through understanding, inspiration. e.g.,reasons, details, answers. The "why, how, Got it!"	Replenisher of spirit.
ATTITUDE: ILLUMINATING THE LIFE FORCE "Let it Shine, Shine, Shine LET IT SHINE." (Adverse Reaction: Mood swings, scattered, hyper, anxiety.)			

ZEN-TOUCH™ MERIDIAN ASSOCIATIONS. FUNCTIONS, RESPONSES, ATTITUDES

FUNCTION	Physical	Emotional	Mental/Philosophical
HEART REGULATOR: Emotional Regulator, "Gateway" Protects through regulation	Regulates intake of blood to heart. "Buffers"	Regulates magnitude of emotional reception. Gateway to heart.	Regulates intake of inspirational fuel. Tempering intensity spiritual fire.
TRIPLE HEATER: Emotional circulator/transporter	Regulates heat production and its destination.	Transports healing power of emotional fuel.	Transports or inhibits spiritual fuel to upper, middle, or lower body.

ATTITUDE: HARMONIZING THE SOULS INSPIRATION.
Maintains constancy and durability. (Adverse Reaction: Faded charisma - dull "cold".)

FUNCTION	Physical	Emotional	Mental/Philosophical
SPLEEN/PANCREAS: Focus and endurance. The resources to initiate focus and "follow through."	Governs stamina, evenness of energy level through blood sugar, mineral and white blood cell management.	Bonding, generosity, nurturing, safety, compassion — regulates the glue, thread, connection to relationships.	Provides our, 1) universal awareness, 2) creative power and, 3) our inspirations with, 4) *a down to earth* reality. Nourishes "Soul."
STOMACH: Tempo or pace of "following through."	Digestive activator, governs our physical pace of carrying out metabolic functions.	Resonance and connection with others in carrying out of desires. Drives the pace of our focusing.	Collective spiritual motivation. Community Drive.

ATTITUDE: I AM HERE BY CHOICE, SAFE AND CONNECTED. PARTICIPATING IN PEACE, I RESPECT ALL. (Adverse Reaction: Over thinking, worry, demanding, blames others.)

FUNCTION	Physical	Emotional	Mental/Philosophical
LUNG: Gathering for completing of self. "Individuation"	Governs energy through respiration, first layer of immune response.	Gathering/collecting heartfelt experiences for understanding of *self* relevance.	Discovering of self, nature, lineage, uniqueness, and style.
LARGE INTESTINE: Eliminating the extraneous.	Elimination of wastes and plays partial role in water balance, and nutrient absorption.	By letting go, we build on the past.	Understanding personal past, and letting go to allow future growth. Soul Enrichment Evolution.

ATTITUDE: I REVERE AND RESPECT "SELF," UNIQUE, WITHIN THE INTERCONNECTION OF THE WHOLE. (Adverse Reaction: Stagnation, stuck, guilt, shame, blame self.)

Our challenges and difficulties materialize for us to improve and develop consciousness. They arise because we have what it takes to transcend them. The associations listed above can identify specific directions to better navigate one's life path. Practitioners can support clients in their journey by becoming an objective witness to the circumstances and energies that are calling for attention.

Motivate and encourage clients who experience fatigue to improve and appreciate the stamina and endurance that their positive attitude, diet, and exercise will provide. Advice and recommendations reap results when a client's spirit is moved.

While knowledge, imagination and compassion are great guides, I find that the practitioner's most valuable skill is the ability to hold a safe space for clients to find their own way. Too many words offered as well meaning advice often bring a client out of the "healing session environment" by stimulating the analytical mind.

Instead Zen-Touch™ practitioners may create affirming poetic metaphors based on the complimentary callings of the client. For example, if a practitioner senses a "restless" feeling in the area associated with future direction (liver) and a barren/untouched sense of loneliness in the "understanding self" (lung) she may create a phrase, connected to the meridian's seasonal image which directs beneficial change.

As Spring winds gently fan and soothe the tension in branches of future growth....the root remembers its unique nature.

[Liver was Full("tension in branches of future growth") its dispersion ("Spring winds gently fan") is poetically suggested.... Lung(" the root") was empty, it now fills ("remembers its unique nature.")]

Phrases like this could be offered to the client for use as an affirmation, or the Zen-Touch™ practitioner simply tunes in to the feeling of the phrase while holding the two areas. Empathizing with the client's energy is highly effective in facilitating change. We hold the space that generates balance.

In class, each student reads a phrase depicting the direction of beneficial change while the others guess which areas were empty or full.

Other Examples:

Phrase: Fire's passion kindles the earth's craving.
Balances: (Heart Full) with (Spleen Empty)

Phrase: Sediments of the past melt away and summer's circulation power is now free to move—high or low.
Balances: (Large Intestine Full) with (Triple Heater Empty)

Phrase: Life awareness, like a winter storm, finds its place and yearning desire is finally satiated.
Balances: (Kidney Full) with (Stomach Empty)

Exercise

Offer explanations for the following, i.e., which area was full and which was empty.

Rocks of Antiquity dissolve to fulfill the need for Destiny's Courage

_____was Full   _____was Empty

Sparks of many possibilities inspire the starving need for safety within.

_____was Full   _____was Empty

Emotion's Door widens its opening and healing circulates to all body zones.

_____was Full   _____was Empty

Safely embraced, worry is transformed, an idea is finally envisioned.

_____was Full   _____was Empty

CASE STUDIES

The following are summarized examples of individual cases, which will provide some practical insight as to how we can connect with our clients' conditions.

CASE STUDY #1

Sheri S. - She begins by talking about her pain in the shoulders and neck. "No one has been able to do anything with this. I've tried everything from painkillers to herbs and acupuncture. No one can get rid of this for me."

Her last statement is the most important factor in her assessment and therapy. She spoke the truth - no one can heal her. She alone wills her own healing. Health practitioners *initiate* changes and provide education.

Assessment and Therapy

Upon working with her, the *gallbladder meridian* in the shoulders and neck was extremely tight and stiff. The *liver* assessment area in the *back* was very *Full*. The *liver* area in the *Hara* was somewhat expanded or swollen, but the most overall *Full* area was at the bottom of the *descending colon. Kidney* and *Large Intestine* areas in the back were the most *Empty*. Working to move the intestines, through stimulating the legs and Hara, was the most efficient method for generating change. Also, tonifying *Bladder* meridians and the *Kidney* area in the back proved very effective. [An important lesson here is: When many areas reveal imbalance, focus on the place(s) that respond(s) most to therapy. These are the assessment areas that are *presently* most receptive to change and will yield the greatest benefits. *Therapy* becomes the *assessment.*]

Intuitive Assessment

I sensed that she never felt nurturing with her father during her youth. She later revealed that she was never loved by her father because of the resentment he held toward his wife. Social implications kept him in the marriage. Sheri was their only child and believed she was the only reason that he remained married.

Confirmation of Lifestyle with Body Condition

Her insecurity in youth created a longtime pattern of *fear* that she would never experience love (*kidney* back area - *Empty.*) She has resented her father since youth and she has yet to *"let go"* of this (*Large Intestine Full* in the *Hara*). Her weakness in the back area (*Kidney* and *Large Intestine - Empty*) stemming from youth, created a situation where her intestines were sluggish. Holding on to this past influence gives her an excuse of why her life development has been impeded. Physically, the *Liver* is forced to overwork to balance the stagnation in the *Kidneys* and intestines, while she holds the *"rising"* tension in her upper back and shoulders. The source seems to be lower in the body. (*Kidneys EMPTY & Large Intestine FULL.*)

Perhaps she believes no one, except for her father, can cure her. While psychological understanding and transformation is very important, it is equally important she strengthen the involved organs through diet, exercise, and nurturing bodywork. This practical approach will initiate clear thinking and the transformation of her psychological stagnation.

CASE STUDY #2

Jack C. - Jack has *"sciatica"* (pain along the sciatic nerve, which runs down the back of the legs). He is a recovering alcoholic. His energy is low in mid-afternoon.

Assessment and Therapy

Liver is Full in the Hara and in the legs. Spleen/Pancreas meridian is Empty in the legs and Hara, but Full and very tight in the Back assessment area. The Bladder meridian in the legs is tight and highly receptive to deep stimulation with elbows.

Therapy consists of relaxing bladder meridian in the legs, tonifying spleen meridian and sedating liver energy. A more vegetable-based diet will transform the buildup of animal fats from the past. Stretching bladder meridian in the legs and self-massage in the Hara are effective recommendations for him to do at home. Support from friends and his recovery group are encouraged to foster a sense of safety and connection.

Intuitive Assessment

Jack's desire for freshness and spontaneity are the most important desires his body is calling for. Closer relationships at home and the pursuit of his deeper dreams and visions will support this craving.

Confirmation of Lifestyle with Body Condition

Perhaps Jack's past alcohol abuse caused the glycogen storage capacity in the liver to be exceeded. The excess was deposited as fat in the buttock area. When he is feeling pressured, his body contracts and the result is pressure on the sciatic nerve = pain! For a long time, his pancreas has been very tight, (SP/PA area — Full in the Back — perhaps from too much animal food and salt). This physically contracted situation made him crave expansion from alcohol. This extreme pattern may have weakened his body's blood sugar regulation. Thus, he gets tired in mid-afternoon when the sun is descending (Earth SP/PA energy).

CASE STUDY #3

Benjamin D. - Ben came in wearing a bright orange jumpsuit. His face was broken out in a rash and he complained of itching on his legs (liver and spleen meridian) and fatigue. He was an actor and displayed what I considered to be an incredibly magnetic and very witty personality.

Assessment and Therapy

In the legs, Spleen meridian was extremely Empty, and Liver was very Full. In the back, Liver area was extremely hard and Full and Heart area was very hard and armored.

The overall therapy involved tonification in all Empty areas. Great nurturing was necessary. Advice centered around simplification of lifestyle to better focus on his health. Important daily disciplines necessary to initiate results included: more root and ground vegetables in his diet, to initiate strength and focus; moderate exercise (strenuous exercise might cause excess mineral loss); deep breathing and meditation.

Intuitive Assessment

Ben's flamboyance is a guise for some deep pain related to rejection at an early age.

Confirmation of Lifestyle with Body Condition

The overall assessment suggested an acid blood condition from which bacterial infection (skin challenges) and fatigue result. His fire-like personality manifested in such a way that Ben found it difficult to focus on grounding his life. In terms of the Five Transformations, he burned every bit of fuel and left himself with insufficient reserves to carry out his goals (excess fire, inhibiting metal). Because the Large Intestine was compromised, his skin acted as an outlet for discharging waste (skin eruptions and itching). His lack of energy could be traced to a lack of minerals held for reserve in the Spleen. A compromise in the Spleen was most likely affecting his lymphocyte production, thus leaving his immune system requiring fortification.

Benjamin commented about his fear of rejection. Small, courageous steps in sharing intimacy will be embraced more easily in supportive surroundings from his closest friends.

◆

One of the most important principles of Health Assessment is that every indication be observed in relation to the person it manifests in. For example, two people may suffer from a headache, however, the cause and therapy for that headache may be completely different for each person.

When we place the emphasis of our therapy on the person, instead of the indication, we will learn that every person is unique. The possibilities for change and healing are therefore infinite and each client becomes a teacher, as we understand the dynamics of his unique life situation.

When working with someone, make observations and then let them go. As we work with our clients, the most relevant information will re-materialize. If an overly analytical approach pervades, we may miss the forest for the trees. Experience is our best guide. The more people we work with, the more we will be shown very practical and intuitive lessons.

This holistic approach to healing, although abstract and oftentimes illusive, provides an opportunity to cultivate human perception and intuition.

CULTIVATING OUR HEALTH

Cultivating sound health will support vitality of body, mind and spirit for the practitioner and everyone he or she works with. The body could be compared to a sensitively charged antenna wire, receiving and transmitting energy to assist clients in the quest for health, happiness, and harmony.

The following sections will address some of the basic methods available to us for cultivating vitality.

POSTURE

Posture is very important in enhancing and circulating energy. A slouched or tense body can limit our potential to initiate successful therapy. Bodily freedom assists the mind to remain clear and receptive throughout the session. If we are stiff and inflexible, or lethargic and disconnected, that feeling will be communicated in our work.

Maintaining a relaxed, yet connected, posture initiates powerful flowing energy in a session and prevents the possibility of picking up any stagnated energy that might be released by the client.

Poor posture can be compared to a bent garden hose. When the bend is straightened, water surges through. When our body alignment is straight, our energy flows freely.

"A Clear vessel connecting and channeling universal life force."

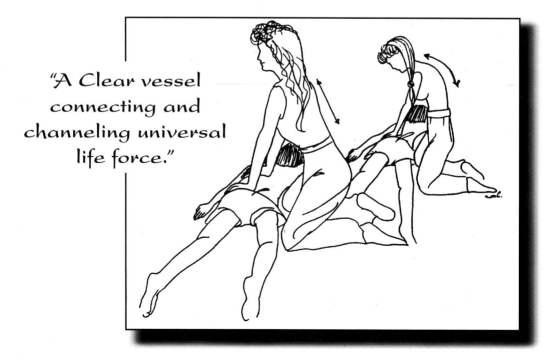

Figure 50

EXERCISE and BREATHING

The circulation of blood, lymph, and internal energy initiated through body movement makes some form of daily exercise essential to our wellbeing. Regardless of ones body structure, or dis-ease, all pain and ailments can be alleviated or prevented when the circulation of energy is activated and flowing freely. An exercise program that suits each person's condition can be a tremendous benefit.

One of the most effective ways to stimulate energy movement is through deep diaphragmatic breathing. Breathing in this manner expands the lungs to their full capacity, enhancing all metabolic functions. It can be incorporated as part of any exercise and eventually becomes a natural breathing pattern that maintains vitality while initiating a calming body disposition. As a practitioner, deep breathing during sessions keeps us centered and greatly diminishes the possibility of picking up negative influences discharged by clients.

The following diagram illustrates a simple and very effective breath circle exercise that I recommend practitioners utilize during sessions.

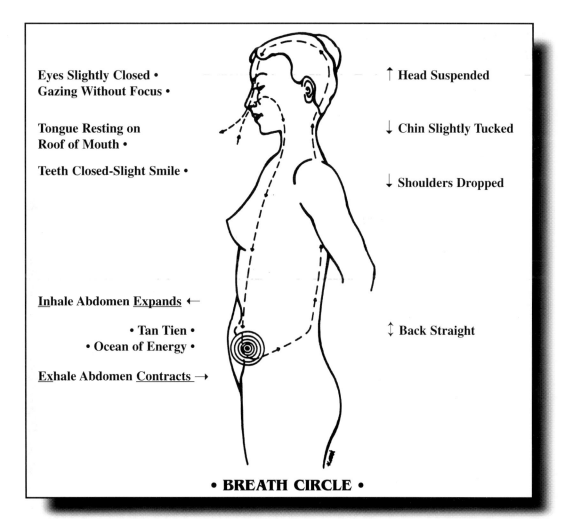

Eyes Slightly Closed •
Gazing Without Focus •

Tongue Resting on
Roof of Mouth •

Teeth Closed-Slight Smile •

↑ Head Suspended

↓ Chin Slightly Tucked

↓ Shoulders Dropped

Inhale Abdomen Expands ←

• Tan Tien •
• Ocean of Energy •

Exhale Abdomen Contracts →

↕ Back Straight

• BREATH CIRCLE •

Figure 51

This is actually a very natural and powerful breathing system. Most babies and animals do it automatically. Many people forget this instinctual breathing method as they grow older and replace it by breathing shallowly, utilizing only chest and upper lung movement. When we inhale deeply, we activate our lungs from top to bottom. This complete breath action pushes on the diaphragm under the rib cage and in turn expands our abdomen, thus stimulating all our internal organs. Most martial arts and yoga forms utilize deep diaphragmatic breathing.

When working with clients, deep diaphragmatic breathing serves to charge the body, thus keeping the practitioner in a state of great vitality. Also, it is very important to move with the client's body as they breathe. For example, if she or he is exhaling, then this is the best time to shift our weight forward. As they inhale, we shift our weight back. This pattern is very natural, and either client or practitioner can introduce it at any time in a session, either verbally or just through the natural touch communication that is set up during a session.

Many sources recommend that the practitioner follow the client's breath pattern, i.e., both practitioner and client could inhale and exhale in unison. Sometimes this method serves as a great way to connect with the client. However, if the client is a shallow breather, it may prove disadvantageous to the therapy by compromising the vitality of the practitioner. What works very well for me is to move my body in unison with the client's breath pattern, while maintaining my own independent slow and deep breathing pattern. This method maintains a united rhythm between client and practitioner, while simultaneously cultivating an independent vital energetic flow within the practitioner's body.

Most people who develop this slow breathing method report increased focus and vitality in their sessions. They also comment on the ease of remaining safe within "other people's stuff" and being free from "burnout."

FOOD

The most profound dietary concept that influenced me was the understanding that sound nutrition was much more than ingesting a quantitative measurement of nutrients, i.e., counting calories and observing recommended dietary allowances. The expression, "you are what you eat" has continued to provide a basis for understanding that the quality of food we eat translates into the quality of our blood and all body cells.

I would like to suggest that it is much easier for practitioners to initiate clear, energizing, transformational work when they are nurturing themselves through one of our most basic requirements: food. Every individual has different dietary requirements and there are many dietetic concepts to choose from.

The study of yin and yang and Eastern philosophy led me to "Macrobiotics." This is a system of balancing food according to the principles of *yin/yang* and the *Five Transformations*. It addresses individual health supporting requirements relating to different lifestyle, geographical and climatic conditions.

Macrobiotic's principles go hand in hand with the system that Shiatsu is based upon, e.g., if a person is manifesting an overly *expanded or contracted* behavior pattern which parallels with one of the *Five Transformations*, a complimentary dietary change will support the client in her transformation to health.

If you are interested in further Macrobiotic studies, I recommend books by George Ohsawa, Michio and Aveline Kushi, and Herman and Cornelia Aihara. I also have written *Food for Life* a handbook primer on the subject. A list of recommended reading and reference books is included at the end of *The Art of Zen Touch*™.

MEDITATION

Meditation traditionally means "sitting quietly." Many methods have been developed to create this state of quiescence. The purpose of meditation is to clear the mind of distracting thoughts and create a deep receptive state where energy from the universe flows freely through the body. In this state our bodies become physically, emotionally, and spiritually nourished.

Many practitioners develop themselves through such practice. When we feel clear and focused we can similarly initiate this feeling with our clients. The meditative state also opens our consciousness to the deeper perspectives of our lives and the lives of the people we work with.

Persistent Chaos
Running through my brain…
A breath of wind, a gentle stream
A drop of Rain
- Sitting in Silence…An opening
- A millisecond of space
- A vacuum - Troubles forgotten
Clear of Blame
Ahh…Quiescence -
Bubbling Blood, Rippling from my veins - creating
peace
Whole Again
                                                        SK

Ideally, the work itself becomes a meditation. The postures, breathing, nutrition and quiescence of the mind that we bring to our sessions make our work a health promoting activity. How wonderful to be involved in a profession that cultivates better health and improves our lives.

ATTITUDE

A common attitude in bodywork is that practitioners have a responsibility to "heal," or at the very least, make things better. Placing too great a responsibility on ourselves often gets in the way of our ability to effect positive change. The word I have used so often is "initiate." If we think of ourselves as initiators, or catalysts, as opposed to doers or healers, the responsibility of change is shifted to the client. We can thus facilitate and support changes in those clients who are ready and willing to change. The practitioner is less like a personality and more like an environment that inspires clients to change.

Although it would be nice to initiate benefits with everyone we work with, in reality this situation is rare. A different style of bodywork, practitioner, or therapy alternatives may offer a client beneficial healing and changes. Attachment or responsibility to achieve results inevitably drains the practitioner. Let's compassionately support our clients in any direction they are motivated to move.

In the actual session, stay clear, minimize thoughts, breathe deeply and follow intuition as to how and where to work. Milton Trager called this state of mind "hookup." Some have described it as "channeling." Whatever we choose to call it, communicating with our clients in this spontaneous meditative fashion works wonders. Once we have learned a number of techniques, and we are comfortable using them, we can then focus solely on openly perceiving which techniques work for each client and session. Eventually, new techniques will be spontaneously generated from our bodies, and we will be shown how to best work in the *Present*…the greatest *Gift*.

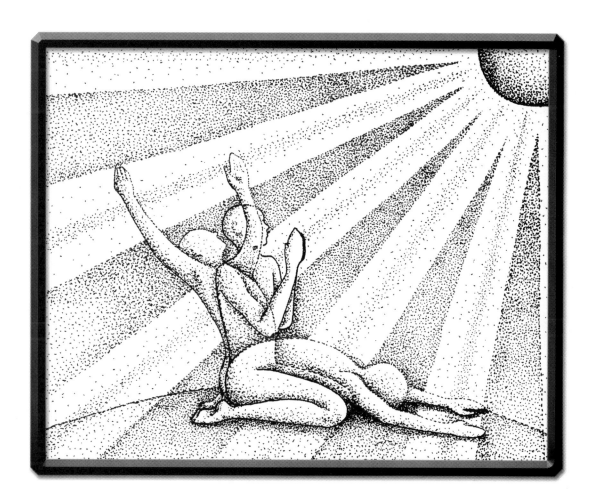

ZEN-TOUCH™ MOVES

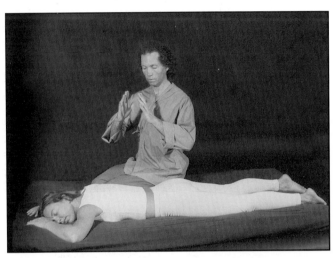
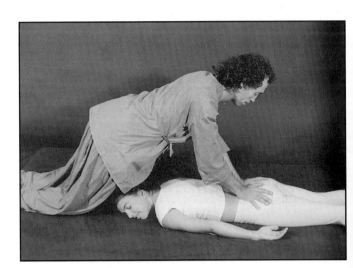
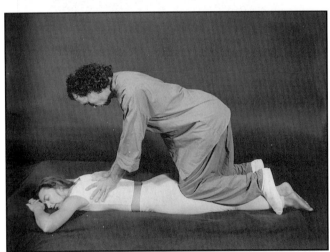
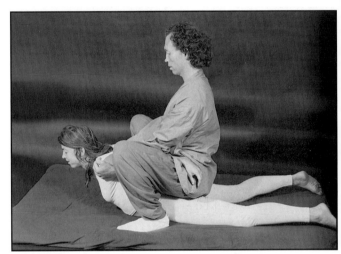
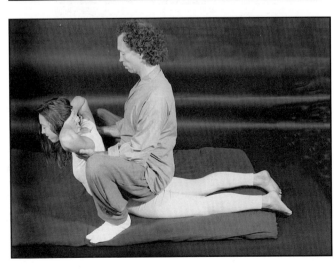
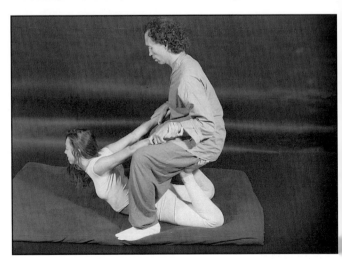

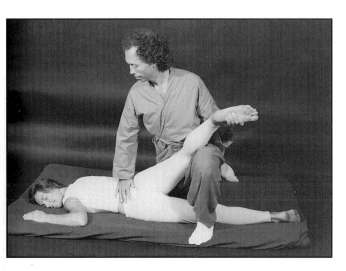
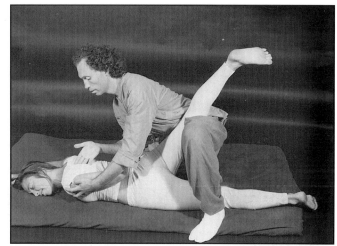
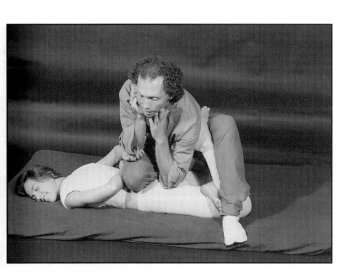
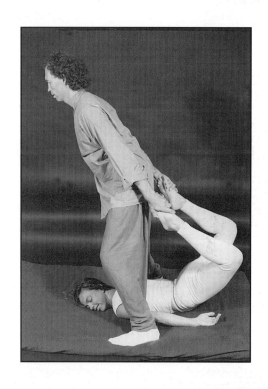
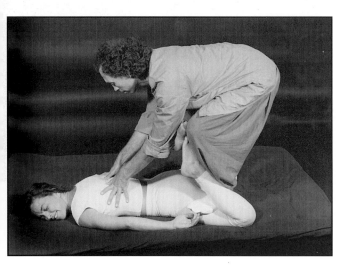
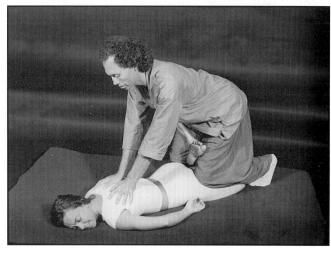

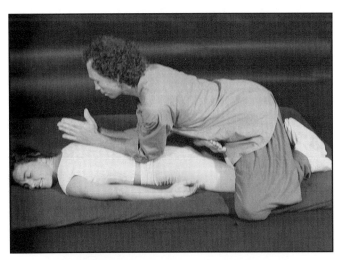
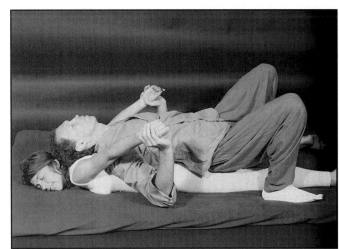
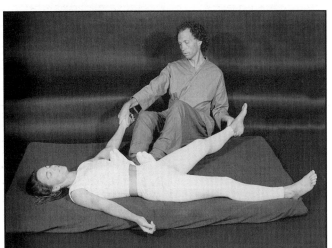
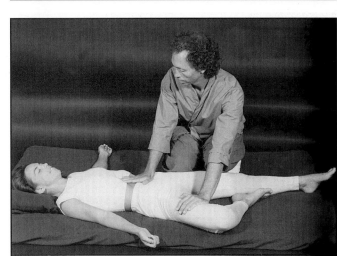
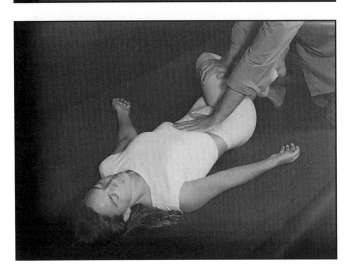
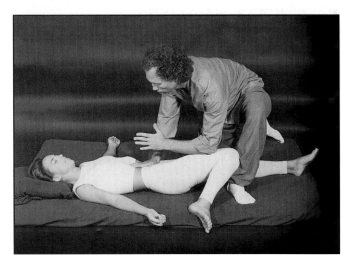

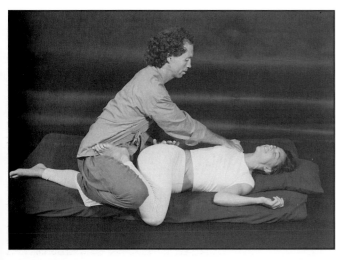
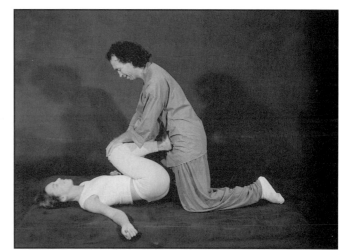
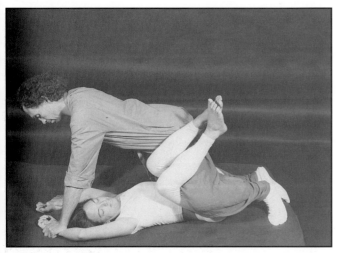
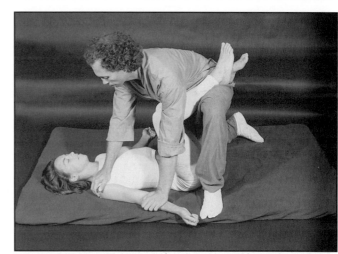
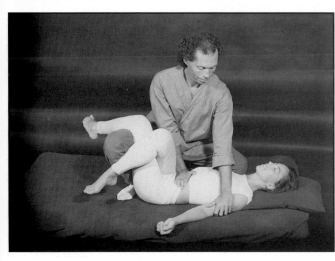
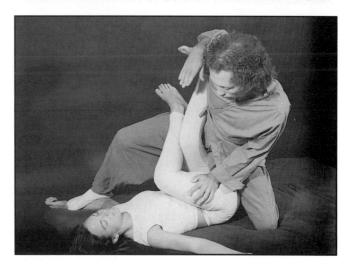

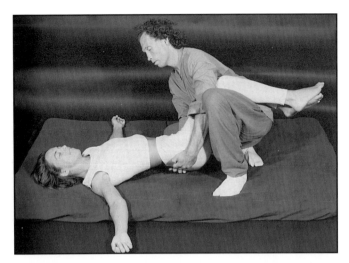
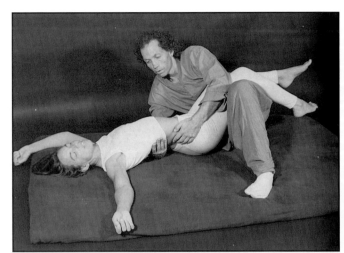
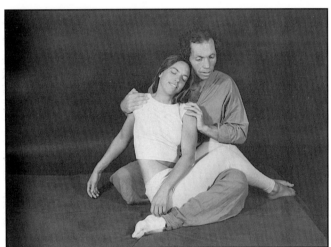
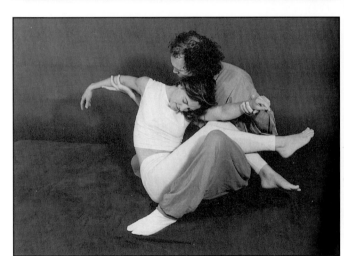
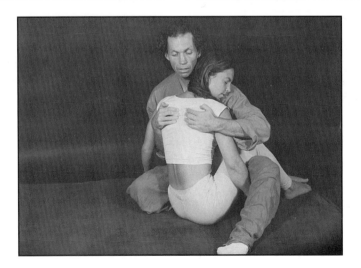

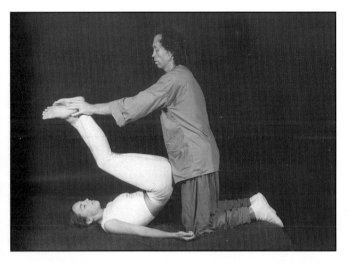
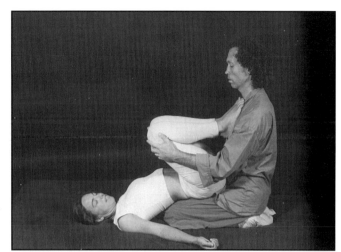
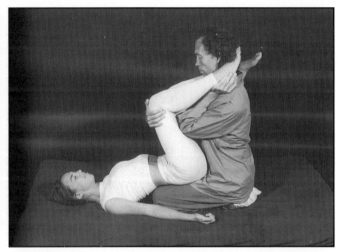
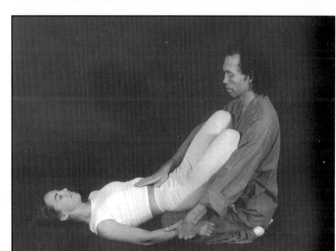
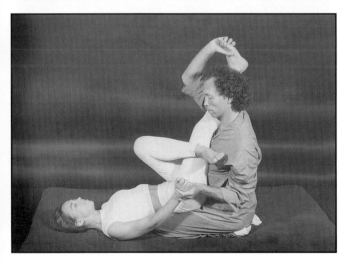
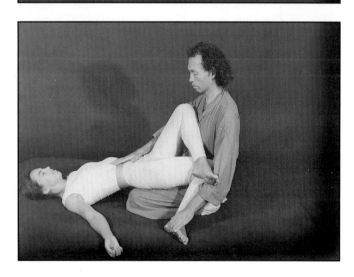

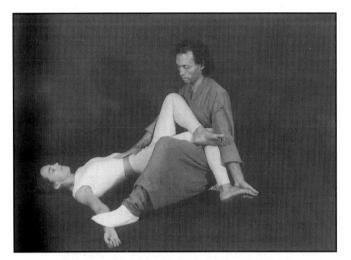

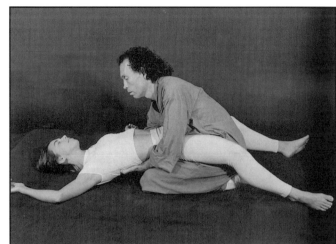

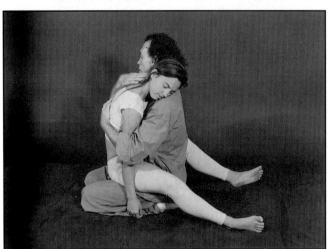

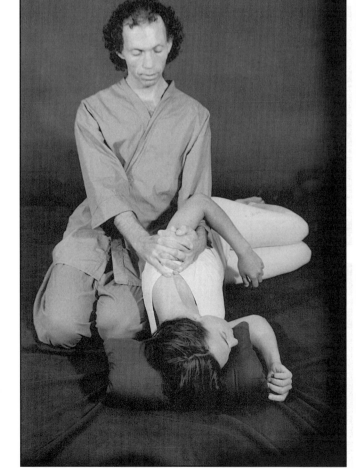

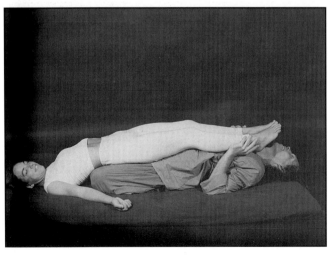

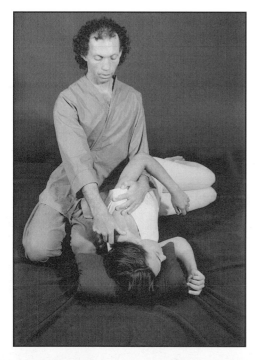
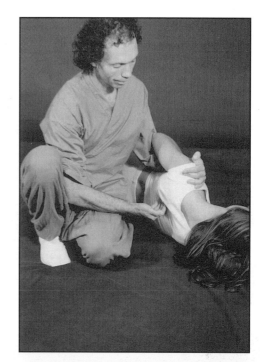
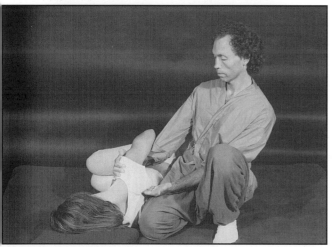
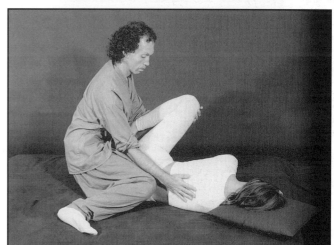
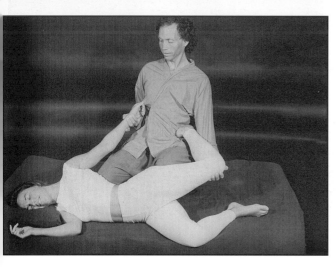
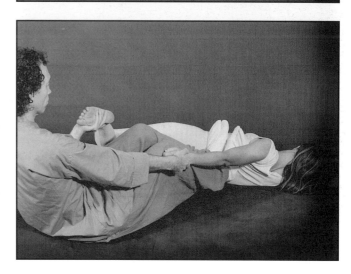

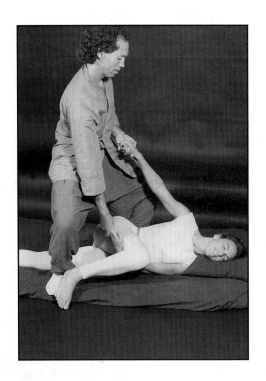

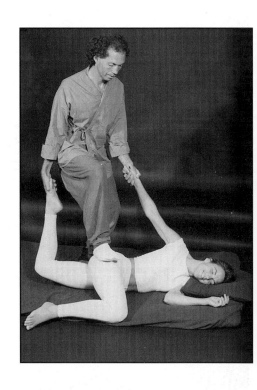

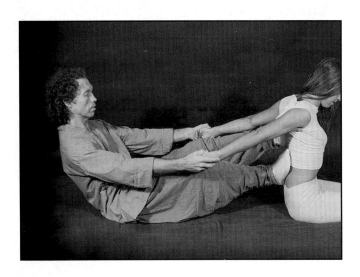

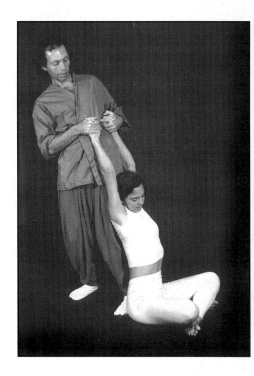

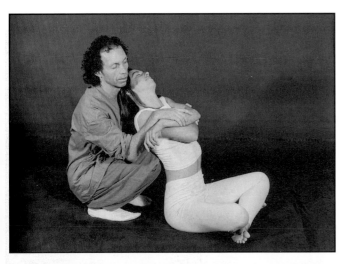
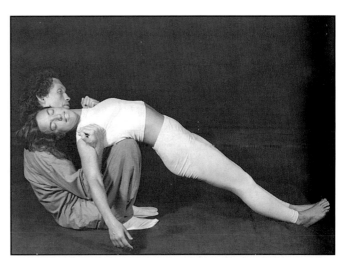
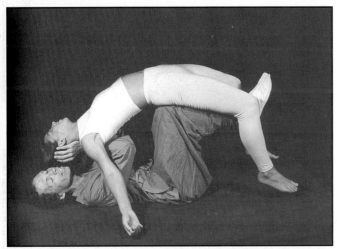
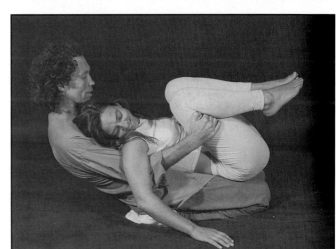
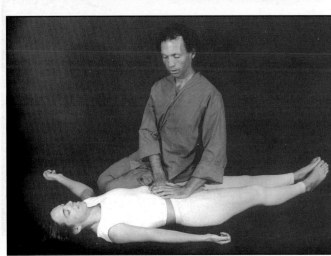
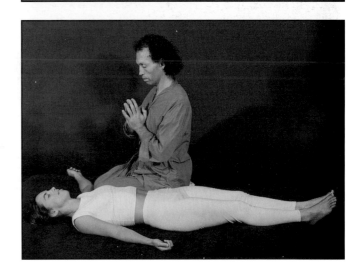

Knowledge, Imagination, Compassion and Intuition are great guides, and of course, experience will fine-tune our approach when working with different individuals.

"Work with hands alone…a Mechanic.
Work with hands and head…a Craftsman.
Work with hands, head, and heart…an Artist."
Work in Emptiness…Magic."

———————— ◆ ————————

Each person a symphony
One movement…the next
A sombrous ode
A magnificent crest
Subtly sweet, torrentous rain
Ride the wave of balance
That mysterious terrain
Trust the moment – Slow…perhaps soft…
or Direct and Bold
The story unfolds, the puzzle is blessed
In the touch of compassion Health is caressed.
Zen-Touch™~ Moves

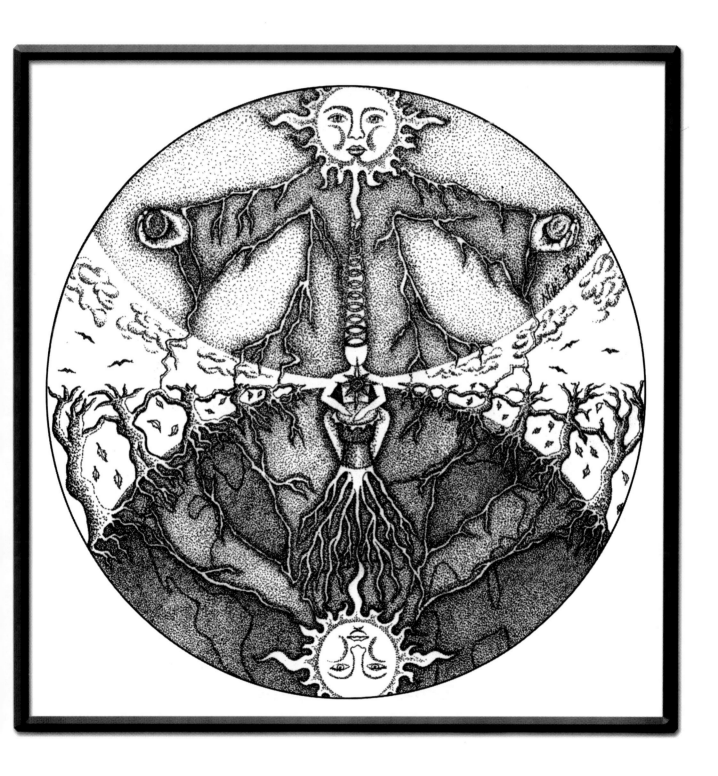

REFERENCES
AND RECOMMENDED READING

Do it Yourself Shiatsu, by Wataru Ohashi

Zen Shiatsu, by Shizuto Masunaga

An Outline of Chinese Acupuncture, by Chinese Academy of Traditional Medicine

Acupuncture Medicine by Yoshiaki Omura

Barefoot Shiatsu, by Shizuko Yamamoto

Family Health Care, by Shizuko Yamamoto & Patrick McCarty

The Book of Macrobiotics, by Michio Kushi

The Book of Oriental Diagnosis, by Michio Kushi

Your Face Never Lies, by Michio Kushi

Macrobiotics and Human Behavior, by Bill Tara

Chinese Face Reading, by T. Mar

Tai Chi Chuan: Principles and Practice, by Master C. K. Chu

Nei Kung, by Master C. K. Chu

Food for Life, the Macrobiotic Approach to Achieving Personal Balance,
     by Seymour Koblin and Janet Lobody

*Shaping Our Destiny - Body Reading & Recommendations for Health,
     Love & Life Path,* by Seymour Koblin

For class/workshop inquires or purchases of Seymour's books, music, educational audio and video tapes call:
(858) 581-9460
www.schoolofhealingarts.com or www.soulstarcreations.com

Index